Understanding Medicinal Plants
Their Chemistry and Therapeutic Action

THE HAWORTH HERBAL PRESS®
Titles of Related Interest

Concise Handbook of Psychoactive Herbs: Medicinal Herbs for Treating Psychological and Neurological Problems by Marcello Spinella

Herbal Medicine: Chaos in the Marketplace by Rowena K. Richter

Botanical Medicines: The Desk Reference for Major Herbal Supplements, Second Edition by Dennis J. McKenna, Kenneth Jones, and Kerry Hughes

Tyler's Tips: The Shopper's Guide for Herbal Remedies by George H. Constantine

Handbook of Psychotropic Herbs: A Scientific Analysis of Herbal Remedies for Psychiatric Conditions by Ethan B. Russo

Understanding Alternative Medicine: New Health Paths in America by Lawrence Tyler

Seasoning Savvy: How to Cook with Herbs, Spices, and Other Flavorings by Alice Arndt

Tyler's Honest Herbal: A Sensible Guide to the Use of Herbs and Related Remedies, Fourth Edition by Steven Foster and Varro E. Tyler

Tyler's Herbs of Choice: The Therapeutic Use of Phytomedicinals, Second Edition by James E. Robbers and Varro E. Tyler

Medicinal Herbs: A Compendium by Beatrice Gehrmann, Wolf-Gerald Koch, Claus O. Tschirch, and Helmut Brinkmann

Anadenanthera: *Visionary Plant of Ancient South America* by Constantino Manuel Torres and David B. Repke

Understanding
Medicinal Plants
Their Chemistry
and Therapeutic Action

Bryan Hanson, PhD

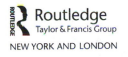

NEW YORK AND LONDON

First Published by

The Haworth Herbal Press®, an imprint of The Haworth Press, Inc., 10 Alice Street, Binghamton, NY 13904-1580.

Transferred to Digital Printing 2010 by Routledge
270 Madison Ave, New York NY 10016
2 Park Square, Milton Park, Abingdon, Oxon, OX14 4RN

AUTHOR'S NOTE
This book explains the chemical and pharmacological principles needed to understand how medicinal plants affect the human body. It has been written with the utmost care as to accuracy, but as an introductory work it is deliberately incomplete from a technical perspective. Although historical and current information about particular plants is given, this book is not intended as a guide to the use of medicinal plants. Before using any medicinal plant product, you should educate yourself about that particular plant and product in detail. Any information that you do not understand should be clarified before use of the product. Consultation with your regular physician or other trusted health care provider is strongly recommended. Neither the author nor the publisher is responsible for the consequences of the use or misuse of information contained in this work.

Originals of the woodcut illustrations were generously made available by the Lloyd Library and Museum, Cincinnati (www.lloydlibrary.org). Images were digitized by Celene Hawkins. Individual illustrations are shown with their sources.

Some figures were prepared using data from the Protein Data Bank (PDB), a government-funded depository of biomolecular data: Figure 4.7 is based upon PDB file 2AAI; Figure 4.9 is based upon PDB file 1BNA; and Figure 6.13 is based upon PDB file 1L0V. Figure 7.16 is based upon the model of Redinbo, Stewart, Kuhn, Champoux, and Hol (1998) published in *Science* 279: 1504-1513.

Cover photographs by Bryan A. Hanson. The plant shown is blood flower (*Asclepias curassavica* L.) photographed at the Wilson Botanical Gardens in Costa Rica by the author.
Cover design by Jennifer M. Gaska.

Library of Congress Cataloging-in-Publication Data

Hanson, Bryan Abbott, 1959-
    Understanding medicinal plants : their chemistry and therapeutic action / Bryan Hanson.
      p. cm.
    Includes bibliographical references and index.
    ISBN-13: 978-0-7890-1551-8 (hc. : alk. paper)
    ISBN-10: 0-7890-1551-X (hc. : alk. paper)
    ISBN-13: 978-0-7890-1552-5 (pbk. : alk. paper)
    ISBN-10: 0-7890-1552-8 (pbk. : alk. paper)
    1. Materia medica, Vegetable—Popular works. 2. Medicinal plants—Popular works. 3. Botanical chemistry—Popular works.
    [DNLM: 1. Plants, Medicinal—chemistry. 2. Phytotherapy. QV 766 H251u 2005] I. Title.

RS164.H276 2005
615'.321—dc22

2004024495

CONTENTS

ABOUT THE AUTHOR

Bryan Hanson, PhD, is the Julian Professor of Chemistry at DePauw University in Greencastle, Indiana, where he has taught for seventeen years. His advanced education includes a bachelor's degree in biochemistry from California State University, Los Angeles, and a PhD in chemistry from UCLA with a focus on the total synthesis of natural products. After two years of postdoctoral work with Jim White at Oregon State University, he began teaching at DePauw in 1986. Professor Hanson's research interests are in the areas of medicinal plants, natural products, and chemical ecology. His primary teaching responsibilities are in organic chemistry, biochemistry, and a course intended for nonscientists called "Medicinal Plants for Poets."

Preface

The idea for this book originated with a course I recently designed and began teaching called Medicinal Plants for Poets. The course is intended for nonscience majors, including those who are "science avoiders" and those who are taking the course only because someone *forced* them to take *something* in the sciences. When I first taught the course it was certainly a delight, but I discovered that no texts or books of any kind addressed the scientific material I wanted to cover and the audience that sat before me. Thus the idea for this work was born.

So exactly who is the audience for this book? Naturally, students in my course and similar courses are the prime audience; this book provides the necessary chemical background to support courses about medicinal plants that range in perspective from botanical to cultural and historical. And, naturally, people who want to know more about medicinal plants should read this book (and a lot of people who use medicinal plants should know more!). But what *kinds* of people might want to read this book? I believe that a wide range of people who are intrigued by science will find this book interesting—the kind of people with a natural curiosity that makes them always want to know a little more. If you regularly or even occasionally pick up a copy of *Scientific American* or *Discover* and read some of the articles, then you are probably going to enjoy this book. Because so many scientific disciplines contribute to our knowledge of medicinal plants, people who know a little about many fields, and especially those who enjoy drawing connections between different fields, are ideal readers of this book. If you consider a book that exercises your mind to be pleasure reading, then this is a book for you.

Writing this book was a great excuse to read more deeply on many interesting topics, and this has enriched me as a scientist. My own training is in organic chemistry and biochemistry, with some pharmacology thrown in on the side. Questions about nature have always interested me, and I find attractive the insights that these fields provide. I have chosen a career in teaching at a liberal arts college, where critical-thinking skills in varied contexts are emphasized. All of these aspects come together in this book; it's primarily a guide to thinking critically about medicinal plants.

Although this book is not intended as a consumers' guide by any means, once you have read this book you will be a lot more savvy about interpreting the claims you hear about medicinal plants and their actions on the human body. *Understanding Medicinal Plants* is not intended to be comprehensive but rather to convey some of the fundamental chemistry, biology, and pharmacology needed to understand the molecules in a medicinal plant and how they can affect your body. I try to get the basic information out there quickly and then explain why understanding a concept is important. As a check and reinforcement, I apply these concepts to actual cases. I want you to know what the important questions are and have some basic conceptual answers to these questions. I've carefully chosen some suggested readings and placed them at the end of selected sections for those of you who want to follow up on a particular topic.

Anytime one writes about a technical subject—especially one that touches on several scientific disciplines—the challenge is to balance rigor with readability. *Understanding Medicinal Plants* aims for the middle ground between a technical publication which assumes its reader is highly trained and a book for the popular press which oversimplifies the material. Although I have limited the depth of many topics, all of the information I have provided is factually sound, and I've tried to avoid simplifying in such a way that it misleads. What you learn in this book can safely be used as a basis for further learning, and I hope that's just what you'll do.

I've tried to draw out the beauty inherent in these complex topics in an accessible, user-friendly way. When you are done reading, I hope you will feel that I have achieved this goal. If the notion of beauty in complexity seems strange, consider the following quote from E. O. Wilson, a highly respected Harvard professor, champion of biodiversity preservation, and author of numerous books:

> The cutting edge of science is reductionism, the breaking apart of nature into its natural constituents. The very word, it is true, has a sterile and invasive ring, like a scalpel or catheter. Critics of science portray reductionism as an obsessional disorder. . . . Practicing scientists, whose business is to make verifiable discoveries, view reductionism in an entirely different way: It is the

search strategy employed to find entry points into otherwise impenetrably complex systems. Complexity is what interests scientists in the end, not simplicity. Reductionism is the way to understand it. *The love of complexity without reductionism makes art; the love of complexity with reductionism makes science.*[1]

This *is* a book about science; in fact, it's about some of the most complex sciences working together to teach us about medicinal plants. If you don't already, I hope you will learn to love the pleasure of teasing understanding out of complexity, and be stimulated to dig deeper on various topics.

NOTE

1. Edward O. Wilson, *Consilience: The Unity of Knowledge* (New York: Knopf, 1998), p. 54, emphasis added.

Acknowledgments

Writing a book is a considerable undertaking that goes much more smoothly with the support of interested colleagues, as well as students who challenge you to make things just a little clearer. I am fortunate to know all sorts of helpful people, and thanks are due to several individuals. Early encouragement on the project was provided by my occasional collaborator Mike Flannery of the Lister Hill Library of Medicine at the University of Alabama at Birmingham. I am grateful to Dave Roberts of DePauw for his assistance in preparing quality space-filling style figures and to Robin DiRocco for assistance in preparing the bibliography. My son Keith Hanson selected the terms for the glossary and drafted the initial definitions. Keith, Kit Newkirk (a friend with a lifelong interest in medicinal plants), and Maureen Bonness (a fellow educator in the field of medicinal plants) carefully read drafts and provided much needed guidance. I am also thankful for the not-always-subtle feedback received from the students in several offerings of my Medicinal Plants for Poets class who used various drafts of the book along the way. Kyle Danforth, using his keen eye, undertook the tedious task of checking all of the chemical structures for accuracy. A great deal of research was necessary to provide the latest information, and Bizz Steele and Angie Battin of the interlibrary loan office at DePauw University were exceptional at locating and promptly providing the many references I sought. Other important resources were provided by the able staff of the Lloyd Library in Cincinnati. The Faculty Development Committee at DePauw provided both funding and time for the writing, which made reasonable progress possible. Finally, I greatly appreciate the helpful editors and staff at The Haworth Press. Thanks to all!

Chapter 1

Introduction

Almost all aspects of life are engineered at the molecular level, and without understanding molecules we can only have a very sketchy understanding of life itself.

Francis Crick

Interest in alternatives to modern medicine has never been higher than it is now, and a large part of that interest revolves around the use of medicinal plants. One can purchase a wide variety of herbal products at virtually any drugstore or all-purpose retailer. Television and magazine ads proclaim the virtues of garlic, ginkgo, and ginseng. You probably know people who regularly use herbal supplements, and you may have used them yourself.

If you have picked up this book and read this far, you are probably the kind of person who has, at one time or another, wondered exactly how drinking an herbal tea can help prevent cancer, or how taking *Echinacea* capsules can help you beat a cold.[1] Perhaps you have heard that red wine and dark chocolate can help prevent cardiovascular diseases such as heart attacks and strokes, and have wondered how such a wonderful thing is possible—though most people don't need excuses to enjoy wine and chocolate!

If so, then you are asking the very questions scientists ask, and how to think about these questions and understand the answers is the subject of this book. Let's look at a common example to illustrate what I mean. Almost certainly you have heard of the plant St. John's wort, which is recommended for the treatment of mild depression. Some of

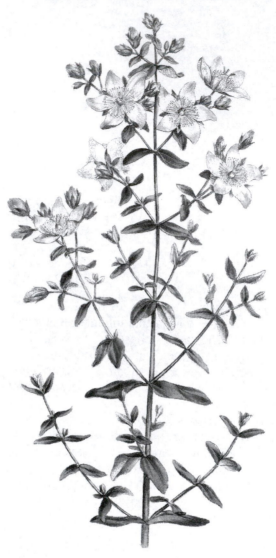

Hypericum perforatum. (*Source:* Woodville, William. *Medical Botany* containing systematic and general descriptions, with pl.s of all the medicinal plants, indigenous and exotic, comprehended in the catalogues of the material medica; as published by the Royal College of Physicians of London and Edinburgh; accompanied with a circumstantial detail of their medicinal effects, and of the diseases in which they have been most successfully employed. London: printed and sold for the author by J. Phillips, 1790, Vol. 1, pl. no. 10.)

the questions you and scientists of various ilk might ask about this plant include the following:

- Does St. John's wort actually treat depression?
- How can I identify St. John's wort when I see it?
- What time of year should I collect the plant?
- What part of the plant should I collect?
- How much of the plant should I take, and how should I take it?
- What are the active ingredients in the plant?
- How do the active ingredients work?
- Can I overdose or poison myself by taking too much?
- Can the plant be dangerous if I'm pregnant or have high blood pressure?

The detailed answers to these questions would require the expertise of a number of different types of scientists:

- Physicians and statisticians would determine if the plant is actually effective in treating depression.
- Botanists would help with the identification of the plant.
- Pharmacologists and chemists would help determine what time of year and what plant part to collect, as well as help the physicians with dosage issues.
- Chemists would isolate and identify the active ingredients.
- Chemists, pharmacologists, physiologists, and perhaps molecular biologists would help us figure out how it works.
- Toxicologists and physicians could take this information one step further to help us understand whether the plant might poison us or have side effects.

As you can see, with all these "-ologists," the study of medicinal plants is a busy field (academics call it interdisciplinary). Still other scientific fields might be relevant: ethnobotanists and anthropologists to help interpret the medicinal plant knowledge of other cultures, pharmacognocists[2] who would contribute in a variety of ways, and so on.

I'm certainly not prepared to discuss all of these areas, but I point them out to illustrate the nature of medicinal plant investigations. In fact, the previous questions only scratch the surface, as St. John's wort has other interesting properties besides being an antidepressant. Regarding its antidepressant activity, however, scientists are still not completely certain which molecule is responsible. For many years it was thought that the antidepressant activity of St. John's wort was due to a molecule called hypericin, though now other molecules are under consideration (see Figure 1.1). My point is that even after identifying hypericin (or anything else) as an active ingredient, scientists will have many more questions, such as how to analyze a plant or a pill for its hypericin content.

So this book is about *questions* about medicinal plants, particularly questions about what's in them and how they work—in other words, *understanding* medicinal plants. It is intended for nonscientists, and I have tried to write for this audience. I have tried to maintain rigor but keep the writing accessible through careful explanation and careful choice of examples. *Understanding Medicinal Plants* is not the place to find information about specific herbs for particular medical conditions; many books about that topic are already available. Rather, my goal is to provide a basic knowledge of the concepts and principles needed to understand what kinds of molecules are in a medicinal plant and how they exert their influence on the human body. This may be everything you want to learn about right now, but should you eventually want to investigate a particular plant further, you will have an excellent foundation so that you can ask the right kinds of questions, and understand the answers. Although this book is about how to think about and understand medicinal plants, what you will learn can be applied to any molecules used as drugs, whether they come from a plant, a fungus, a bacterium, or even a pharmaceutical company's laboratory.

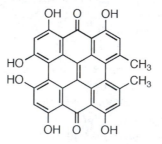

FIGURE 1.1. Hypericin, a molecule found in St. John's wort *(Hypericum perforatum)*.

Understanding Medicinal Plants is organized as follows. In Chapter 2 we will learn to interpret the symbolism of chemical structures, such as the diagram of hypericin in Figure 1.1. These diagrams often scare people away from further reading on chemical topics, so it is well worth the time to try to demystify it. We will also talk about the naming of molecules and consider the enormous range of chemical structures that are possible.

In Chapter 3 we will look at just enough background on chemical bonding that we can begin to understand molecular properties such as the shape of a molecule. Shape turns out to be critical in understanding how a drug works on a molecular level, so we must have some appreciation of this area.

Chapter 4 is a catalog of sorts, in which examples of the different chemical families found in plants are given. This is good information to browse through at first and turn to later when more specific information on a particular family is needed (or it can be skipped entirely).

Chapter 5 looks at chemical behavior that is relevant to medicinal substances obtained from plants. We will examine acid-base behavior and such techniques as spectroscopy to see how they can be used to help isolate and identify substances from plants. Then we will turn to exploring the antioxidant properties of medicinal plants, which will bring us back to chocolate and red wine.

Chapter 6 discusses how plant drugs and toxins move through the body and act on specific molecules. We will first look at some general principles that affect how a drug is absorbed, distributed through the body, and eventually excreted in some form. We will then move to a molecular view of what happens once a drug reaches its final place of action (referred to as its target). Material covered in the earlier chapters will be essential to understanding these sections.

Finally, in Chapter 7, we will look at several case studies of medicinal plants and apply all we have learned to understand how these plants work. With the possible exception of Chapter 4, you'll probably want to read the chapters in order.

Before we launch into this material, however, I feel I would be misleading you if I didn't mention something about my beliefs about medicinal plants, because they color my approach to the topic. The word *beliefs* has a religious air about it and, indeed, many people believe that medicinal plants have some special, mystical properties because they are natural, or organic, or God given. For similar reasons, some

folks reject anything considered a "chemical" because they believe
them to be fundamentally bad, or they reject mainstream medicines
because they are synthetic. Indeed, we have much to learn about medicinal plants; in some cases whole herbs, as opposed to extracts or
purified materials, *are* better. But is also true that nature contains
many, many toxic substances, so we should not label plants and natural, herbal treatments as superior in all cases. Like it or not, virtually
everything in the world is a chemical or is composed of chemicals. In
fact, the entire point of this book is to help you think about these kinds
of issues and use your knowledge effectively.

The eminent pharmacognocist Varro Tyler liked to point out that a
great percentage of conventional modern medicines actually come
from plants, and he argued convincingly that "rational herbal medicine is conventional medicine" (Robbers and Tyler, p. 15). In other
words, while many people consider herbs to be alternative medicine,
they really are quite conventional when you examine history and current practice. Tyler also identified ten criteria that are characteristic of
what he called "paraherbalism," which he considered a pseudo-
science. If the difference between rational herbalism and paraherbalism interests you, and I hope it does, be certain to see the introduction
to his book *Herbs of Choice* for more information (details are given in
the suggested reading).

I'd like to briefly emphasize one other concept that should be kept
in mind at all times. The art of healing is complex and multifaceted.
In any culture, healing practices are part psychological and symbolic,
part physiological. Psychological and cultural influences on healing
are fascinating topics and important to understanding the use of medicinal plants, both historic and modern. Much has been written on
these topics, and I hope you have or will read some of the fine works
available. In this book, however, the focus is on the physiological actions of medicinal plants. My hope for you, the reader, is that by
learning some of the chemistry and pharmacology of medicinal
plants, you can move toward a deeper understanding of how to
evaluate what you hear about medicinal plants.

SUGGESTED READING

Balick, M. J. and Cox, P. A. (1997). *Plants, people, and culture: The science of
ethnobotany.* New York: Scientific American Library. A very readable descrip-

tion about how plants affect culture, and how we Westerners "discover" medicinal plants.

Blumenthal, M., Goldberg, A. and Brinkmann, J. (eds.) (2000). *Herbal medicine: Expanded Commission E monographs.* Boston: Integrative Medicine Communications. This is an excellent source to begin digging into individual herbs on a more technical level.

Robbers, J. E. and Tyler, V. E. (1999). *Tyler's herbs of choice: The therapeutic use of phytomedicinals.* Binghamton, NY: The Haworth Herbal Press. One of the best books about what herbs to use for what conditions; also discusses paraherbalism and rational herbalism.

Sumner, J. (2000). *The natural history of medicinal plants.* Portland, OR: Timber Press. A potential companion to this book which presents a botanical/ecological perspective.

Chapter 2

Interpreting the Symbolism of Chemical Structures, or, Finding Your Way Around a Molecule

It is a pity that most people think a scientist is a specialized person in a special situation, like a lawyer or a diplomat. To practice law, you must be admitted to the bar. To practice diplomacy, you must be admitted to the Department of State. To practice science, you need only curiosity, patience, thoughtfulness, and time.

A. Holden and P. Morrison, 1982
CrystalsandCrytalGroing,   p. 11

Many people find chemistry intimidating, and much of that feeling comes from the extensive symbolism used in the field. By symbolism I mean the formulas and structures and everything conceptual that is implied by them (there's a lot of symbolic math in chemistry too, but we won't worry about that). We encounter signs and symbols all the time, but they are familiar. We cease to think about them; we just react. Our system of traffic signs is one example of symbols with specific meanings and implications. Fail to stop at a stop sign and you might hit another vehicle, but we hardly think about this—we just do it.

With a little information and practice, your understanding of chemical symbolism can be developed to this same level. In the Introduction, I showed you the structure of hypericin. To the chemist, a great deal of meaning and information is present in that structure. Also, some degree of abbreviation is used, in that not everything is shown—the viewer is expected to apply certain rules and infer parts of the structure that are not explicitly drawn. Since molecules are the basis of the action of medicinal plants, we need to understand what these symbolic diagrams (chemical structures) mean.

THE BASIC RULES OF BONDING

Before we can examine the meaning of chemical structures, we'll need to know some rules for connecting (bonding) atoms together. For now, we'll ignore how or why or when such bonding occurs and instead concentrate on the symbolism.

You've probably seen the periodic table before and know that many elements have been discovered. Fortunately for us, only four elements are seen regularly in medicinal substances found in plants. They are shown in Table 2.1. The atomic symbol is an abbreviation which is found in the periodic table, and it is used in chemical structures to indicate the location and type of atoms present (we'll look at the periodic table a bit later). One of the simplest ways to remember the bonds that these atoms make is to know the following pattern:

$$1 - 2 - 3 - 4$$
$$H - O - N - C$$

That is, hydrogen (H) makes one bond to another atom, oxygen (O) makes two bonds, and so forth. This memory device seems a bit like a cheer or a chant.[1] Perhaps you can fit it to a tune.

So, we have to keep in mind that any carbon atom, for instance, should make four bonds, at least in the circumstances we'll encounter. I must add that bonds can be single, double, or triple bonds. As you might expect, a triple bond counts as three of the four bonds that a carbon atom can make. It turns out that carbon is the main element in

TABLE 2.1. Important elements.

Element	Atomic symbol
Hydrogen	H
Oxygen	O
Nitrogen	N
Carbon	C

the living world. Figure 2.1 illustrates some of the arrangements that can result when carbon is bonded to other atoms according to the rules we've just given. Note that in the figure, the end of each line should be thought of as connecting to an unspecified atom.

WHAT DO THE LINES MEAN?

Chemists have several different styles of drawing molecules, and at times it seems as though they mix and match styles just to keep you guessing. However, if we know the rules of bonding and a few other facts, we can readily interpret what is meant by any structure. In a chemical structure, a line represents a bond between two atoms. Single, double, and triple bonds are possible, as just mentioned, and one, two, or three lines are used to convey this information. The atom itself may be represented by either its atomic symbol, or by the intersection of two lines, or by the end of a line. In the latter two cases, the atom is assumed to be a carbon atom. If one of these "assumed" carbon atoms appears to have less than four bonds, the missing bonds are taken to be to hydrogen atoms that are not drawn in explicitly. The structure of hypericin is shown again in Figure 2.2 annotated to illustrate these different drawing styles.

With additional effort, we might have drawn out every atom (this is shown in Figure 2.3 and can be called an expanded structural drawing), but chemists are generally a lazy lot,[2] and *do* draw lots of structures, so usually the simpler version is drawn. But when you see the structure in Figure 2.2, you must think in your mind of the structure in Figure 2.3. By studying these structures, you can verify the rules of bonding that were just introduced.

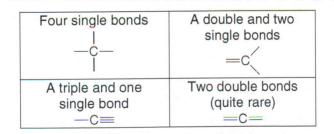

FIGURE 2.1. Common bonding situations for carbon.

A single bond between two carbons

A double bond between two carbons

A carbon atom with four bonds to other carbon atoms (one is a double bond)

An oxygen atom with two bonds

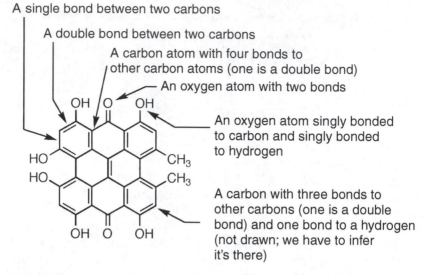

An oxygen atom singly bonded to carbon and singly bonded to hydrogen

A carbon with three bonds to other carbons (one is a double bond) and one bond to a hydrogen (not drawn; we have to infer it's there)

FIGURE 2.2. Interpreting the chemical symbolism in the hypericin drawing.

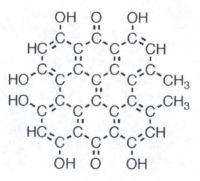

FIGURE 2.3. The expanded (and time-consuming) style of drawing structures.

At times, you might see structures represented in still other ways. For example, in Figure 2.4, note how the top –CH₃ group on the right side of the molecule has been replaced by a line. Since a line that ends without an atomic symbol is considered to be a carbon atom, and it has only one bond drawn in explicitly, we can use the rules of bonding to infer that there must be three hydrogens on that carbon atom (that's

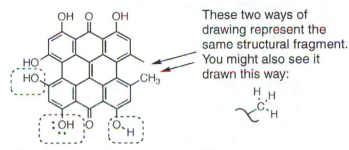

The three boxed areas represent the same functional group, but the bottom left box with its electrons drawn in conveys additional information that is important in certain circumstances.

FIGURE 2.4. More on how to interpret the symbolism.

what the subscript 3 in "$-CH_3$" tells us too). Thus, the two ways of drawing are equivalent. We eventually will need to know more about this symbolism (e.g., the electrons I slipped into Figure 2.4), but I hope you are getting more comfortable with chemical structures. We'll get plenty of practice in the next few pages.

RECOGNIZING THE FUNCTIONAL GROUPS

Nearly every molecule contains what chemists call functional groups. A functional group is a collection of atoms bonded together in a particular way. They are the focus of reactivity in the molecule. Further, under the right circumstances, a functional group in one molecule might attract a functional group in another molecule. Understanding this is very important to understanding how a drug might interact with a protein, for example (which we'll cover later, in Chapter 6). So, we need to be able to recognize the functional groups when we see them.

Many functional groups are possible, but once again, our lives are made simpler because not all of them are relevant to molecules found in plants. Table 2.2 lists the functional groups by their name, and gives several different ways that people write and abbreviate their

TABLE 2.2. Common functional groups.

Name	Structure	Shorthand
Alkane	See text	See text
Alkene	$R_2C=CR_2$ (drawn)	R_2CCR_2
Alkyne	$R-C{\equiv}C-R$	RCCR
Alcohol	$R{-}O{-}H$	ROH
Ether	$R{-}O{-}R$	ROR
Amine	R_3N (drawn as R–N–R with R)	R_3N
Ketone	$R{-}C(=O){-}R$	RCOR
Aldehyde	$R{-}C(=O){-}H$	RCHO
Carboxylic acid	$R{-}C(=O){-}O{-}H$	RCOOH or RCO_2H
Ester	$R{-}C(=O){-}O{-}R$	RCOOR or RCO_2R
Amide	$R{-}C(=O){-}N({-}R){-}R$	$RCONR_2$
Nitrile	$R-C{\equiv}N$	RCN

structures. One of your first questions after looking at the table is probably, "What the heck does that R mean?" By now you probably realize that it too is more symbolism. In this case it represents a placeholder that we use when we don't need to, or don't want to, specify exactly what is attached. Most of the time we should take R to mean a carbon atom with some other atoms attached. In any case, R is assumed to make only one bond to whatever it is attached.

I did not include the structure of the alkanes in the table because we need to discuss them a bit more. Alkanes are the simplest carbon-based molecules; they are composed of carbon and hydrogen only and are connected by single bonds only. This restriction still leaves many possible structures and thus no one structure I could put in the table would properly represent the alkanes. You could say that the characteristic feature of the alkanes is actually a lack of other functional groups, which means they shouldn't be in the table at all. However, we use the alkanes as sort of a reference point, so I them in the table anyway. The alkanes are also known as the saturated hydrocarbons; because they have only single bonds, they have the maximum amount of hydrogen per carbon atom. The other hydrocarbon groups would be considered unsaturated, which is another way of saying they have double or triple bonds in their structure. Note that in the table I shaded the alkanes, alkenes, and alkynes to remind us that they are all types of hydrocarbons.

I should add that another group of hydrocarbons exists which I left off the table. As a group, these are called the aromatic hydrocarbons; you can recognize them because the molecule benzene is their building block.[3] Benzene is a ring of six carbons with alternating double and single bonds; it is shown in two drawing styles in Figure 2.5.

If you look back at the structure of hypericin (Figure 1.1), you should be able to see four aromatic rings hidden in there (benzene is a particular compound, so when benzenelike rings are seen in structures as building blocks, it is best to call them aromatic). I didn't put aromatics in the table because they are not really a functional group. However, they are very common, and we will refer to them often, so I thought it best that you hear about them early on. A benzene ring connected to something by a single bond is generally called a phenyl group and is abbreviated Ph or Ar (these are short for phenyl or aryl).

In the real world, of course, molecules are not as simple as Table 2.2 implies. Just about any molecule you encounter would likely have more than one functional group. One skill you ought to have is the ability to look at a molecule and see the functional groups and other features embedded within it. Since you've probably grown weary of

FIGURE 2.5. Benzene.

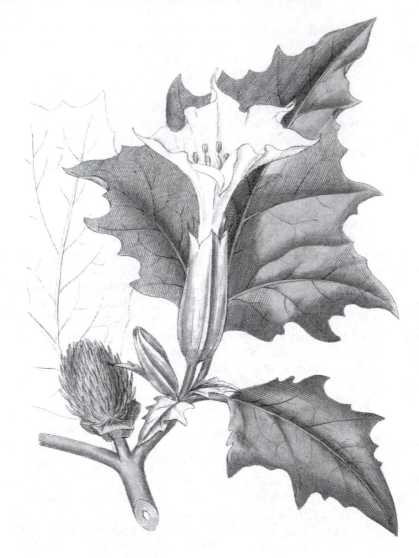

Datura stramonium. (*Source:* Woodville, William. *Medical Botany* containing systematic and general descriptions, with pl.s of all the medicinal plants, indigenous and exotic, comprehended in the catalogues of the material medica; as published by the Royal College of Physicians of London and Edinburgh; accompanied with a circumstantial detail of their medicinal effects, and of the diseases in which they have been most successfully employed. London: printed and sold for the author by J. Phillips, 1792, Vol. 2, pl. no. 124.)

hypericin, let's look at another plant molecule, atropine. As with many other molecules, this one is both useful and toxic. It is found in a plant commonly called jimsonweed or devil's apple (the Latin name is *Datura stramonium*), and compounds within it have important uses in emergency medicine and surgery. The structure of atropine with the functional groups circled and categorized is shown in Figure 2.6. The part of the molecule that is not marked off is an alkane—a hydrogen and carbon framework of single bonds. The majority of molecules you will encounter can be thought of as an alkane framework decorated with functional groups. Since the functional groups are generally the interesting part, we hardly give notice to the alkane part. Hypericin, as it turns out, is an exception to this generalization. The only parts of hypericin that would be considered alkanes are the two $-CH_3$ groups. Everything else is a functional group or an aromatic ring.

As a final example of identifying functional groups, examine the structure of camptothecin (see Figure 2.7), an anticancer compound which also has a number of toxic side effects (the action of camptothecin and its relatives is discussed in Chapter 7). In this structure I have also introduced a new form of symbolism: the use of wedges and dashes to give some sense of the three-dimensional shape of a molecule. We will encounter this form of drawing and learn its full significance later.

NAMING MOLECULES

Now that you've met some molecules, we ought to say something about how molecules are named, because one frequently sees multi-

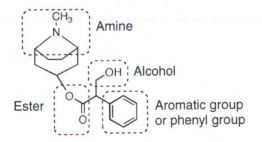

FIGURE 2.6. Atropine with the functional groups labeled.

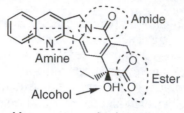

Amide

Amine

Alcohol

Ester

▲ Means a group is closer to the viewer (in front of the paper)

▟ Means a group is farther from the viewer (behind the paper)

FIGURE 2.7. Camptothecin, an anticancer compound.

ple names for the same molecule. Chemists have developed a system for naming molecules referred to as "systematic nomenclature." The basic ideas are fairly simple, or at least systematized, but because molecules get complicated rather quickly, the names do too. A molecule might also be called by its common name, or by a trade name if it is a drug.

For example, you are probably familiar with the pain reliever called Aleve. This is a brand name or trade name. If you have seen a magazine advertisement for Aleve, or bought a generic form of it at the drugstore, you probably encountered another name for the same thing: naproxen sodium. Naproxen sodium is the common name or generic name.

Chemists also need a more complicated name (for some very good reasons which we won't discuss). Whatever you are inclined to call it, the chemists' systematic name for Aleve is sodium (S)-(+)-6-methoxy-α-methylnapthaleneacetate. Obviously this is a mouthful; this name represents yet another kind of chemical symbolism. If you had to say this all the time, you'd quickly come up with an alternative, such as naproxen sodium. If you went to the pharmacy and asked the staff for some sodium (S)-(+)-6-methoxy-α-methylnapthaleneacetate, they probably wouldn't know what you were talking about. It is much more practical to call it naproxen sodium on a day-to-day basis.

In fact, you already know and use common names for many molecules: aspirin, chlorophyll, hypericin, penicillin, and so on. Such names are useful because the chemists' technical names don't exactly roll off the tongue. The systematic name for chlorophyll requires a long paragraph to write out. However, if you wanted to know the chemical structure of Aleve, the brand name is worthless—it tells us nothing about the structure. This is one reason why systematic names exist. If you know the rules, the systematic name tells you how to draw the structure.

The point right now is to realize that naming molecules can be done in several ways, each with advantages and disadvantages. Some are brand names, designed to be easy to remember and catchy, so they sell well. Others are common names, merely a convenience. At times, one might want to—or have to!—use the systematic name, full of information and symbolism.

SAMENESS: MOLECULAR FORMULAS AND ISOMERS

Even before picking up this book you probably knew that many different types of chemicals existed in the world. As we wrap up our discussion of chemical structures and symbolism, we should discuss what makes molecules the *same* or *different* from each other.

To chemists, the concept of "sameness" is very important. We want to be able to compare two structures and determine whether they are the same. We also want to make sure that any difference we see is real, not an artifact of how a molecule is drawn. This can get complicated, so for now we will explore only enough to illustrate the concepts and lay a foundation for the rest of the book.

As a group, molecules that are different in certain ways and the same in others are called isomers (*iso* means equal in Greek), but molecules can be the same or differ in several ways, so we need to narrow our language a bit. For now we will consider what are usually called structural or constitutional isomers, molecules that have the same molecular formula but different connectivity.

The *molecular formula* is simply a list of the atoms in a molecule, with subscripts to indicate how many of each kind there are. For instance, if you added up all of the atoms in the structure of atropine (see Figure 2.6), you would come up with a molecular formula of $C_{17}H_{23}NO_3$. Note that only one nitrogen is present, but we don't write N_1; we simply write N. We also write the formula with Cs first,

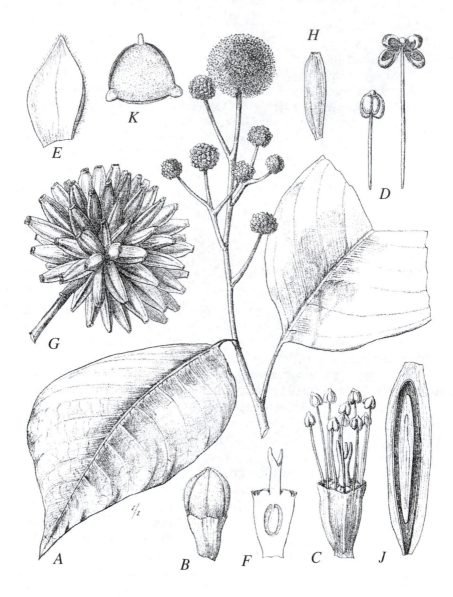

Camptotheca acuminata. (*Source: Das Pflanzenreich: Regni Vegetabilis Conspectus* heraugegeben von. A. Engler. Leipzig: W. Engelmann, 1910. 41. Heft, IV, 56a, Garryaceae, p. 16, fig. 3.)

then Hs, and then any other elements in alphabetical order (out of re-spect for the importance of carbon!). Keep in mind that all but one of the hydrogens in the formula had to be inferred from the structure us-ing the rules of bonding explained earlier; they are not drawn in the structure.

The problem with this formula is that it doesn't tell us much about the structure. (Well, truthfully, it does put *some* limits on the struc-ture, but there are still so many possibilities that it's overwhelming.) We don't know, for instance, which functional groups are in the mole-cule, or where they are, or if any rings are present. If we had the sys-tematic name, we could use it to figure out the structure (but we'd also have to learn all those rules, and even then it would be challenging). The fundamental problem here is that we don't know how the atoms are connected; what I call the *connectivity*. If you had only the for-mula of atropine (and at one time that was all that chemists had), find-ing the structure would be a virtually unsolvable problem. To address this concept in a more manageable way, let's use a simpler example.

Let's say that you had a molecule with formula C_4H_{10}. What are the possible ways to connect these atoms together following the rules of bonding? One good way to answer this is to start drawing. Since the carbon atoms form a framework for the hydrogens (or any other atoms that might be present), think first about how you can arrange and connect the carbon atoms, then add the proper number of hydro-gens. There are only two possible structures that fit this formula; they are shown in Figure 2.8. Note that on the left side of the figure, I used the "lazy" chemists method of drawing. On the right side, I give some equivalent structures with more detail drawn. Remember that we would prefer to use the style of the left-hand drawings but see the style of the right-hand drawings in our mind's eye.

If you tried this problem before seeing the answers, you might have come up with some of the structures shown in Figure 2.9, or oth-ers that are similar. These drawings are equivalent to the first isomer shown in Figure 2.8, because they have the same connectivity. By this I mean that each one is a string of four carbons all in a row along with the associated hydrogens; no branching is present (the second isomer in Figure 2.8 is a string of three carbons with a fourth carbon attached to the middle of the string; this is called branching). It is important to realize that the four structures in Figure 2.9 are different ways of

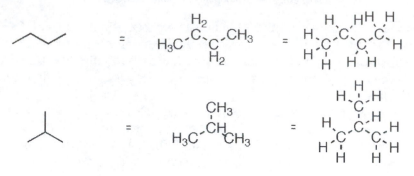

FIGURE 2.8. The two C_4H_{10} isomers drawn in various styles.

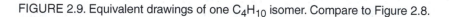

FIGURE 2.9. Equivalent drawings of one C_4H_{10} isomer. Compare to Figure 2.8.

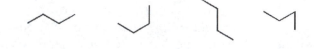

FIGURE 2.10. Different C_4 compounds.

drawing the same thing. We don't want to mistake a different way of drawing something for a truly significant difference.

On the other hand, the two structures in Figure 2.10 *are* different from each other, even though they look very similar. In the left-hand structure, the carbons are bonded together to form a ring. In the right-hand structure, the carbon atoms are in an open chain. If you count the hydrogens in each structure you will see that they are different in this way too (which necessarily follows from the presence of the ring).

One can continue this exercise of translating formulas into structures with different connectivities essentially forever. Even if we stick with just the alkanes (hydrocarbons with only single bonds, which is what C_4H_{10} is), the possibilities are huge, as seen in Table 2.3. As you can see, even if we consider only structures arising from differences in connectivity, and restrict ourselves to the alkanes, the number of

TABLE 2.3. Formulas and the isomeric possibilities.

Formula	No. of isomers possible
C_5H_{12}	3
$C_{10}H_{22}$	75
$C_{20}H_{42}$	366,319

structures quickly becomes unmanageable. What if you were asked to draw the structure of $C_{17}H_{23}NO_3$? The practicing chemist would have the very same problem you would. There are just too many possible ways to connect these 44 atoms. What if this wasn't a "thought" experiment but a real one, and you were given a bottle of a chemical labeled $C_{17}H_{23}NO_3$? Given enough time, you might be able to draw all the *possible* structures, but only one would be atropine. Unfortunately, the drawings don't tell you what is actually in the bottle. To see how we might find out which possible structure is right, you'll have to wait until we get to Chapter 5. For now, I want you to see the nature of the problem: A formula simply isn't enough to specify a single structure from the many that are possible, and *many* are possible.

SUGGESTED READING

Hoffmann, R. (1997). *The same and not the same.* New York: Columbia University Press. An excellent and provocative discussion of what makes things, including chemicals, the same or not. Also considers the concept of purity, and "natural" versus "unnatural."

Le Couteur, P. and Burreson, J. (2003). *Napoleon's buttons: How 17 molecules changed history.* New York: Tarcher/Putnam. A very readable discussion of industrial and medical molecules which by their invention and discovery determined the course of history. Written by chemists, it emphasizes how small changes in structure give rise to rather different properties. About half of the 17 molecules are of medicinal, psychoactive, or nutritional interest. Highly recommended.

Chapter 3

The Origins of Bonding and Molecular Properties

In Chapter 2 we explored how to interpret the symbolism of chemical structures. We now will delve into a fuller background for the basis of that symbolism. It is, after all, a symbolism communicating information about real objects—molecules. So, we need to know how and why atoms bond together. Then we can consider how the structure of a molecule can tell us about its properties, which in turn will tell us about the molecule's behavior as a drug. Bonding and molecular properties are thus essential to understanding everything else in this book.

ELEMENTS, ATOMS, AND THE PERIODIC TABLE

Atoms of different elements are the fundamental building blocks of all matter, including molecules of medicinal interest, so we should spend some time discussing these building blocks before using them to create molecules.

An element is a substance that cannot be separated into simpler substances by a chemical reaction.[1] This is a nice textbook definition, although rather impractical in many ways (e.g., how do you know if you have tried all possible chemical reactions?). Perhaps it is better to think of it this way: if something is not an element, it must be a compound, which is a combination of two or more elements. A compound, in contrast to an element, *can* be broken down further. Examples of elements are the oxygen you are breathing, the carbon in the pencil you use (although it suffers the misnomer "lead," a different element), and the aluminum in aluminum foil. Applying our definition using aluminum as an example, we would say that a sample of aluminum foil cannot be broken down any further and still be aluminum.

On the other hand, water (H_2O) serves as an example of a compound. With the appropriate conditions, we can break water down further, into hydrogen and oxygen gases, which are themselves elements.[2] Other simple compounds that most people are familiar with include carbon dioxide (CO_2) and alcohol (as found in liquor –C_2H_6O).

Let me be clear: It is possible to break apart an element, but if you do so you will no longer have the element—it will be destroyed. In such cases, you are breaking the individual atoms down into neutrons, protons, and electrons, which are almost the smallest known bits of matter (the neutrons and protons are found in the center of the atom, which is the nucleus; the electrons are found outside the nucleus).[3] Atoms are the smallest pieces (particles) of an element that have the properties and behavior of that element, such as a certain melting point or the ability to react with another element. As a definition this too is rather impractical, because until recently no one had ever devised an experiment to see a single atom of something, much less determine whether it behaves as our theories predict. It may seem strange that scientists create definitions that are untestable, but there are certain conceptual advantages to doing so. These definitions are summarized in Figure 3.1.

The most useful information scientists have learned about the elements is contained in the periodic table of elements. The periodic table provides a means of organizing a large amount of information gathered over more than 100 years. It provides the scientist with both a way to remember things and a means of drawing analogies. It also reveals important information about how the elements combine with one another, which enables the periodic table to tell us about compounds as well as the individual elements.

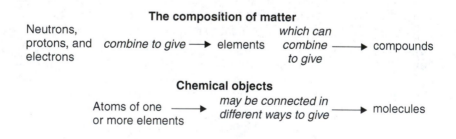

FIGURE 3.1. Definitions related to composition and objects.

Let's take a brief tour around the periodic table (see Table 3.1) before learning how to apply it to understand bonding in molecules. In each box in the periodic table is the symbol used to represent that atom. (I have also provided a list of the symbols with the full name and atomic number of each element in Table 3.2.) Usually the symbol is chosen in such a way as to help us remember the name of the element, although for some elements the symbol's origin lies in its linguistic history, not its current name. Also in the box is the atomic number. The atomic number is equal to the number of protons in the atom's nucleus, which gives the atom its unique identity. This information will be useful to us later.

Where did the periodic table come from? Chemists, their predecessors (the alchemists), and physicists have been making observations of the elements and their compounds for hundreds of years. These observations include such things as the visual appearance of the elements, their melting points, their atomic masses, and their densities. They also include chemical reactivity, such as acidic or basic character, the ability to react with water, or the formula of the compound formed between a particular element and oxygen or chlorine, for example.[4]

By the 1800s, enough of these kinds of observations had been made and shared with the scientific community that people began to identify patterns in some of these properties, especially if one listed the elements in order of increasing atomic mass. For instance, it was noted that the atomic masses of certain elements were the average of the atomic masses of other elements which shared similar patterns of reactivity. A number of scientists published the patterns they had noticed; such information was used to gradually improve the ideas of those that followed. Credit for the major breakthrough, however, goes to the Russian Dimitry Mendeleyev and the German Julius Lothar Meyer. In 1869 they separately published their ideas which became our modern periodic table. At the time, only 63 elements were known (now they number more than 100), but if they were arranged in columns of increasing atomic mass, rows could be made in which each set of elements in a row had similar chemical and physical properties.

One difference between the periodic table of 1869 and the modern version is the format: the rows and columns of today's version are transposed compared to the original. Also, the modern periodic table orders elements by their atomic number, not their atomic mass. These two numbers parallel each other in most cases, so this is not a significant difference. Mendeleyev's early periodic table is shown in Table 3.3.

TABLE 3.1. The periodic table of the elements.

Legend:
- XX — Atomic number
- M — Atomic symbol
- Transition metals

1	2	3	4	5	6	7	8	9	10	11	12	13	14	15	16	17	18
1 H																	2 He
3 Li	4 Be											5 B	6 C	7 N	8 O	9 F	10 Ne
11 Na	12 Mg											13 Al	14 Si	15 P	16 S	17 Cl	18 Ar
19 K	20 Ca	21 Sc	22 Ti	23 V	24 Cr	25 Mn	26 Fe	27 Co	28 Ni	29 Cu	30 Zn	31 Ga	32 Ge	33 As	34 Se	35 Br	36 Kr
37 Rb	38 Sr	39 Y	40 Zr	41 Nb	42 Mo	43 Tc	44 Ru	45 Rh	46 Pd	47 Ag	48 Cd	49 In	50 Sn	51 Sb	52 Te	53 I	54 Xe
55 Cs	56 Ba	57 La	72 Hf	73 Ta	74 W	75 Re	76 Os	77 Ir	78 Pt	79 Au	80 Hg	81 Tl	82 Pb	83 Bi	84 Po	85 At	86 Rn
87 Fr	88 Ra	89 Ac	104 Rf	105 Ha	106 Sg	107 Bh	108 Hs	109 Mt									

Lanthanide series

58 Ce	59 Pr	60 Nd	61 Pm	62 Sm	63 Eu	64 Gd	65 Tb	66 Dy	67 Ho	68 Er	69 Tm	70 Yb	71 Lu

Actinide series

90 Th	91 Pa	92 U	93 Np	94 Pu	95 Am	96 Cm	97 Bk	98 Cf	99 Es	100 Fm	101 Md	102 No	103 Lr

TABLE 3.2. Atomic numbers, symbols, and names for the elements.

No.	Symbol	Name	No.	Symbol	Name
1	H	Hydrogen	32	Ge	Germanium
2	He	Helium	33	As	Arsenic
3	Li	Lithium	34	Se	Selenium
4	Be	Beryllium	35	Br	Bromine
5	B	Boron	36	Kr	Krypton
6	C	Carbon	37	Rb	Rubidium
7	N	Nitrogen	38	Sr	Strontium
8	O	Oxygen	39	Y	Yttrium
9	F	Fluorine	40	Zr	Zirconium
10	Ne	Neon	41	Nb	Niobium
11	Na	Sodium	42	Mo	Molybdenum
12	Mg	Magnesium	43	Tc	Technetium
13	Al	Aluminum	44	Ru	Ruthenium
14	Si	Silicon	45	Rh	Rhodium
15	P	Phosphorus	46	Pd	Palladium
16	S	Sulfur	47	Ag	Silver
17	Cl	Chlorine	48	Cd	Cadmium
18	Ar	Argon	49	In	Indium
19	K	Potassium	50	Sn	Tin
20	Ca	Calcium	51	Sb	Antimony
21	Sc	Scandium	52	Te	Tellurium
22	Ti	Titanium	53	I	Iodine
23	V	Vanadium	54	Xe	Xenon
24	Cr	Chromium	55	Cs	Cesium
25	Mn	Manganese	56	Ba	Barium
26	Fe	Iron	57	La	Lanthanum
27	Co	Cobalt	58	Ce	Cerium
28	Ni	Nickel	59	Pr	Praseodymium
29	Cu	Copper	60	Nd	Neodymium
30	Zn	Zinc	61	Pm	Promethium
31	Ga	Gallium	62	Sm	Samarium

TABLE 3.2. *(continued)*

No.	Symbol	Name	No.	Symbol	Name
63	Eu	Europium	87	Fr	Francium
64	Gd	Gadolinium	88	Ra	Radium
65	Tb	Terbium	89	Ac	Actinium
66	Dy	Dysprosium	90	Th	Thorium
67	Ho	Holmium	91	Pa	Protactinium
68	Er	Erbium	92	U	Uranium
69	Tm	Thulium	93	Np	Neptunium
70	Yb	Ytterbium	94	Pu	Plutonium
71	Lu	Lutetium	95	Am	Americium
72	Hf	Hafnium	96	Cm	Curium
73	Ta	Tantalum	97	Bk	Berkelium
74	W	Tungsten	98	Cf	Californium
75	Re	Rhenium	99	Es	Einsteinium
76	Os	Osmium	100	Fm	Fermium
77	Ir	Iridium	101	Md	Mendelevium
78	Pt	Platinum	102	No	Nobelium
79	Au	Gold	103	Lr	Lawrencium
80	Hg	Mercury	104	Rf	Rutherfordium
81	Tl	Thallium	105	Ha	Hahnium
82	Pb	Lead	106	Sg	Seaborgium
83	Bi	Bismuth	107	Bh	Bohrium
84	Po	Polonium	108	Hs	Hassium
85	At	Astatine	109	Mt	Meitnerium
86	Rn	Radon			

The Meyer/Mendeleyev periodic table was useful in that it organized many observations into patterns. However, the real strength of their work was its predictive power. Within the chart published in 1869 were empty spaces from which, based upon the patterns, it had been concluded that elements must be missing. By using the patterns of physical and chemical properties of the adjacent elements, Meyer

TABLE 3.3. Mendeleyev's early periodic table.

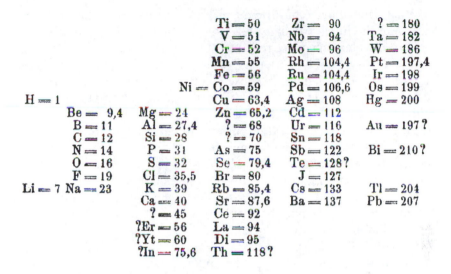

```
                                    Ti = 50    Zr =  90    ?  = 180
                                    V  = 51    Nb =  94    Ta = 182
                                    Cr = 52    Mo =  96    W  = 186
                                    Mn = 55    Rh = 104,4  Pt = 197,4
                                    Fe = 56    Ru = 104,4  Ir = 198
                             Ni = Co = 59      Pd = 106,6  Os = 199
H = 1                               Cu = 63,4  Ag = 108    Hg = 200
        Be =  9,4  Mg = 24          Zn = 65,2  Cd = 112
        B  = 11    Al = 27,4        ?  = 68    Ur = 116    Au = 197?
        C  = 12    Si = 28          ?  = 70    Sn = 118
        N  = 14    P  = 31          As = 75    Sb = 122    Bi = 210?
        O  = 16    S  = 32          Se = 79,4  Te = 128?
        F  = 19    Cl = 35,5        Br = 80    J  = 127
Li = 7  Na = 23    K  = 39          Rb = 85,4  Cs = 133    Tl = 204
                   Ca = 40          Sr = 87,6  Ba = 137    Pb = 207
                   ?  = 45          Ce = 92
                   ?Er = 56         La = 94
                   ?Yt = 60         Di = 95
                   ?In = 75,6  Th = 118?
```

(*Source:* Ueber die Beziehungen der Eigenschaften zu den Atomgewichten der Elemente D. Mendelejeff. *Zeitschrift fur Chemie,* Vol. 12, pp. 405-406 (1869)).

and Mendeleyev were able to predict the properties of the missing elements. Within two decades, three of the missing elements were discovered and investigated by others. They proved to have properties extremely close to those predicted by Mendeleyev and Meyer. Further, the trends in chemical and physical properties were so reliable that Mendeleyev was able to determine that some of the atomic masses of the already discovered elements were incorrect. His corrected values were later verified as well.

The story of the development of the periodic table is one of the best examples of scientific methods in action: making careful observations, assembling those observations into patterns, making predictions, and ultimately verifying those predictions. Even more interesting is the fact that neither Mendeleyev nor Meyer knew the real reasons that the elements behaved according to the patterns they had observed.

ELECTRON CONFIGURATIONS:
THE REAL ORGANIZING PRINCIPLE

What Mendeleyev and Meyer did not know, and could not have known at the time, was that the electrons (negatively charged particles) in the elements were responsible for the patterns of properties and reactivity they had used to organize the periodic table. They could not have known this because electrons were not discovered until nearly four decades later, and their full role in organizing the periodic table was not appreciated until the mid-1920s or so. I emphasize, however, that what they didn't know about electrons did not prevent them from organizing the information they did have in a useful way. In fact, the periodic table eventually provided clues as to its own origins, again demonstrating the power of a good theory.

What Mendeleyev and Meyer needed were the results of what is called quantum mechanics or quantum theory. Quantum mechanics is a particular area of knowledge shared by chemistry and physics that deals with the behavior of electrons. The mathematical foundations of the theory are quite complex. Fortunately, we can jump straight to the important results of the theory.[5]

Quantum mechanics tells us that electrons are found in orbitals. Orbitals are extremely important because they turn out to be the basis for the chemical bonding we are discussing. An orbital is defined as a region in space, around the nucleus of an atom, where an electron is likely to be located. We use the term *likely* because another result of quantum mechanics is that we generally cannot say exactly where an electron is at a given time.[6] We can only speak of the probability or chance of its being in a certain location. Consider as an analogy the chances of locating a friend at a given time. During normal working hours, you would probably find a friend at his or her place of employment. You have no absolute guarantee that he or she will be there, but we might say that you have a 98 percent chance of finding your friend at work. It is the same with electrons. We might make a statement such as "There is a seventy-five percent chance of finding an electron within two hundred picometers of the nucleus," but we cannot say exactly where within that range the electron will actually be found.

The atomic number of an element also tells us about its electrons. It is defined as the number of protons in an atom's nucleus. Since protons are positively charged, and atoms have no charge, there must be the same number of electrons in an atom as there are protons. Thus, carbon, with atomic number six, must have six protons and six electrons. Those six electrons are found in orbitals. As it turns out, several different types of orbitals are possible, and each orbital has certain characteristics—but the details need not concern us. Because we are restricting ourselves to the elements that we see most frequently in plant medicinal molecules (H, O, N, and especially C), we need only deal with what are known as the s- and p-type orbitals.

How are those six electrons in carbon spread around these two types of orbitals? It is not random; some very specific rules are needed to answer this question (these rules are another result of quantum mechanics). The first rule is that any one orbital can hold no more than two electrons. The second rule is that the electrons go into the orbitals in the following order:

$$1s \quad 2s \quad 2p \quad 3s \quad 3p \quad 4s$$

You no doubt noticed something else new in this list. We already said that s and p were different types of orbitals, but what about the 1s, 2s, 3s, and 4s? These numbers are technically called the principal quantum numbers, but we don't need to remember that term. Instead, think of it as the row number in periodic table (rows in the periodic table are also called periods). There are actually three subtypes of p orbitals so, at two electrons per orbital, the p types can hold a total of six electrons.

Let's apply our rules to the element carbon, because it forms the framework of medicinal molecules. Carbon has six electrons. If we put them into orbitals following the rules above, and remembering that up to six electrons can be in the p orbitals, we get

$$1s^2 2s^2 2p^2$$

where the superscript represents the number of electrons in a particular orbital. Note that we only needed to put two electrons into the 2p orbitals, though up to six could have been accommodated. This type of notation is called an electron configuration. Exhibit 3.1 gives the electron configurations of a few other elements generated by applying our rules. If you compare the electron configuration given in Exhibit 3.1 for silicon with the one just given for carbon, you can

EXHIBIT 3.1. Electron configurations of a few elements.

He :   2 electrons $1s^2$

Be :   4 electrons $1s^2 2s^2$

O :   8 electrons $1s^2 2s^2 2p^4$

Ne :   10 electrons $1s^2 2s^2 2p^6$

Si :   14 electrons $1s^2 2s^2 2p^6 3s^2 3p^2$

discover for yourself what Mendeleyev and Meyer didn't know. Columns of elements in the periodic table (also called groups or families) have the same electron configuration for the *last set* of electrons added. Carbon and silicon are in the same family and both end in $s^2 p^2$. Because carbon is in row two, it ends in $2s^2 2p^2$, while silicon, in row three, ends in $3s^2 3p^2$. The last set of electrons added are called valence electrons (or sometimes outer shell electrons). So, we would say that carbon and silicon have the same valence electron configuration (in other words, the same arrangement of their valence electrons in the various orbitals). We could describe it more generally as $ns^2 np^2$ where n is the generic row number. Thinking of it this way focuses our attention on the similarities of these elements.

If you extend this idea, you can see that all elements in the hydrogen family (group) have valence electrons of ns^1: H, Li, Na, K, and so forth; n varies with the row. All elements in the fluorine family (known as the halogens) end in $ns2np5$: F, Cl, Br, I, and At.[7] As we will see shortly, the valence electrons in orbitals are responsible for bonding. A very important "take-home" lesson is that similarities in valence electron configuration are the reason why elements in the same column have similar chemical behavior. For instance, the halogens can be expected to make similar types of compounds because they have similar valence electron configurations. This works out in reality: they are found as diatomic (two-atom) molecules in nature (F_2, Cl_2, Br_2, and I_2), and form a compound with one hydrogen atom that is acidic (HF, HCl, HBr, and HI). Not *everything* is the same for a family of elements, but their bonding behavior is the same, and their other properties follow distinct trends. Remember that observing the types of compounds an element can form was one of the key pieces of information Mendeleyev and Meyer used to develop the periodic table. Now we know that electrons are responsible for that bonding behavior.

BONDING TO CREATE MOLECULES

We can now use what we have learned about the electron configurations of the elements to explain the bonding between atoms that creates molecules. Two kinds of bonds are important to us: ionic bonds and covalent bonds. We'll spend less time on ionic bonds because they are not quite as important to our topic of medicinal plants.

Seeking Nobility: The Formation of Ions

Ions are charged atoms or molecules. For now, we will consider only the case of atoms. If an atom somehow gains electrons, it becomes negatively charged because electrons have a negative charge. If it somehow loses electrons, it becomes positively charged. The important question is, Why might an atom gain or lose an electron? The periodic table provides us with the answer, as well as a way to remember the answer.

The answer lies in the family of elements headed up by helium. This family is known as the noble gases or the inert gases; *inert* means they do not like to react, and *noble* conveys a standoffish attitude. Chemists interpret this lack of reactivity[8] as a sign of great stability. Their stability and reluctance to form bonds meant their discovery was delayed compared to the other elements—and it didn't help that they are quite rare on earth. Because of this stability, chemists conclude that the valence electron configuration of the inert gases, ns^2np^6, is a particularly good one to have. This in turn gives us a way to predict which elements might like to gain or lose electrons to form ions. If an element can gain or lose one or two electrons, and thereby achieve the electron configuration of an inert gas, it should be willing to do so because that configuration represents a very stable state of affairs.

As an example, consider fluorine (F), the head of the halogen family. Fluorine's valence electron configuration is $2s^2 2p^5$. If fluorine gained just one more electron, it would have a valence electron configuration of $2s^2 2p^6$, which is the same as neon's (Ne), and therefore would be considered very stable. But if it gained one electron, it would also be an ion, F^-. So, we would predict that *all* elements in the halogen family would be happy to form an ion with a -1 charge (negatively charged ions are called anions). This is indeed what they do, and they achieve great stability in that form.

Using the same method, elements in the beryllium (Be) family, with a valence electron configuration of $2s^2$, can be expected to *lose* two electrons. If they do so, they end up with the valence electron configuration of helium (He). That configuration would be $1s^2$ (the full electron configuration of beryllium is $1s^2 2s^2$, so losing the last two electrons leaves you with $1s^2$). Thus, beryllium should form a $+2$ charged ion (positive ions are called cations), written Be^{+2}. You can extend this method to many elements, as long as the gain or loss of one or two electrons leaves them with the valence electron configuration of an inert gas. In practice, this means that elements from groups 1, 2, 16, and 17 on the periodic table (see Table 3.1) will readily form ions. These are by no means the only elements that will form ions, but they are the most easily predicted ones.

Ionic Bonding and Ionic Compounds

Ionic bonding is based on the simple notion that opposite charges attract, and that compounds must have no net charge. For the reasons just explained, elements in group 1 form $+1$ ions, those in group 2 form $+2$ ions, those in group 16 form -2 ions, and those in group 17 form -1 ions. With this information in hand, we can predict that a compound formed between potassium (K) and iodine (I) is ionic in nature, and is composed of the ions K^+ and I^-. Its formula will be KI so that the positive and negative charges offset each other. In fact, ionic bonding is often thought of as the *transfer* of electrons between two elements. In the last example, the $4s^1$ electron of K can be thought of as having been transferred to the I, so that the I goes from $\dots 5s^2 5p^5$ to $\dots 5s^2 5p^6$, which is the valence electron configuration of xenon (Xe). This leaves the valence electron configuration of K^+ as $4s^0$, or better, $\dots 3s^2 3p^6$, which is the configuration of argon (Ar).

Thus, both atoms get to be like an inert gas (as you consider this, it helps to have Table 3.1 in view).

In a similar way, you can verify that the ionic compound formed between magnesium and bromine will be $MgBr_2$ because Mg will want to lose two electrons to form Mg^{2+} and it will take two Br^- to offset that charge (remember that in molecular formulas the number of a given atom is shown as a subscript unless it is one). On the other hand, we would not expect any compound to form between the elements sodium (Na) and calcium (Ca) because both of these elements want to form cations. A good rule of thumb to remember is that ionic compounds form between elements on opposite ends of the periodic table, because you find elements willing to form cations on the left side, and elements willing to form anions on the right side.

You can use your knowledge of the periodic table and the typical charges carried by various elements in their ionic states to answer other questions. For instance, let's say you encountered the formula $Ca_3(PO_4)_2$. The symbolism tells us that there are two of the PO_4 units because PO_4 is in parentheses with a subscript of two. What is the charge on the PO_4 unit? You can figure this out by remembering that the Ca will have a charge of +2 because of its position in the periodic table. As there are three Ca^{+2}, the total charge contributed by the three Ca is +6. There are two PO_4 groups, which must contribute –6 in total if the compound is to be neutral. That means each PO_4 group must have a charge of –3 on it. Therefore we can conclude that the PO_4 group is really PO_4^{-3}, even though we know nothing else about the group.

Noble Cooperation: Covalent Bonding

The concept of ionic bonding is often reduced to the simple statement that it involves the transfer of electrons between elements. For covalent bonding, the equivalent simple statement is that it involves the *sharing* of electrons between elements. Sharing of electrons turns out to be a bit more complicated than just transferring them, but again the periodic table will be a great help in remembering things.

Writing Lewis Structures of Atoms

To understand covalent bonding, we need to learn to write the Lewis structures of atoms. A Lewis structure is yet another symbolic way to present information. In this case, it is information that you already know from the periodic table conveyed in a slightly different format. The Lewis structure for an atom is the atomic symbol of the atom surrounded by its valence electrons drawn as dots. It is traditional to think of the electrons as being placed one at a time on the edges of a hypothetical square surrounding the atomic symbol, until you have the correct number of electrons. One dot (representing a valence electron) is placed on each edge of the square until there are four electrons (unless of course there are fewer than four valence electrons). One continues to adds dots representing valence electrons so that there are up to two dots on an edge, until you have added all the valence electrons the atom possesses. Consider bromine (Br) with its valence electron configuration of $4s^2 4p^5$, a total of seven electrons. When written as a Lewis structure, this appears as shown in Figure 3.2. Because we know that the elements in a given family have the same set of valence electrons, we immediately know that all of the halogens (F, Cl, Br, I) have the same Lewis structure as bromine, except for the atomic symbol. In a like manner, once you figure out nitrogen's Lewis structure, then you immediately know that of phosphorous.

Writing Lewis Structures of Molecules: The Octet Rule

Two bromine atoms can combine to give a bromine molecule, Br_2, which is held together by a single covalent bond. A covalent bond is formed by the sharing of two electrons. When we want to represent a covalent bond, the two electrons of the bond are drawn as a single line instead of two dots. The electron pairs which are not used in the bond are still drawn as dots, and are referred to as lone pairs.[9] The formation of the Br_2 molecule from separate bromine atoms, drawn in Lewis structures, appears as shown in Figure 3.3. The principle used in drawing Lewis structures of molecules is that you try to spread the electrons around so that every atom is surrounded by eight electrons.

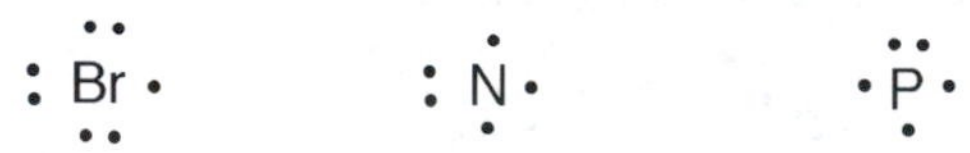

$$\text{: Br :} \qquad \text{: N :} \qquad \text{: P :}$$

FIGURE 3.2. Lewis structures of some atoms.

Figure 3.4 shows the Br_2 molecule again with the counting process (note that we are counting the bonding electrons twice).

Why are we aiming for eight electrons around each atom? This goes back to the inert gases and the periodic table: Each atom wants to have eight electrons around it because the inert gases do, and they are especially stable. This guideline is referred to as the octet rule. The only problem with the octet rule is that there are so many exceptions to it. However, we will only concern ourselves with two of the exceptions. First, hydrogen (H) can accommodate only two electrons around it, so you might say it follows a duet rule. Second, the elements of the boron (B) family are content to have only six electrons, although they are also happy to have eight. Figure 3.5 shows a few more Lewis structures of molecules with only two atoms.

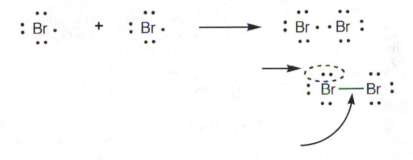

FIGURE 3.3. Formation of Br_2 expressed in Lewis structures.

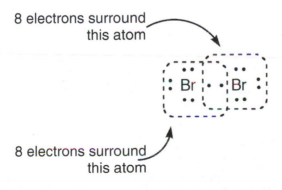

FIGURE 3.4. Electron counting in Br_2.

Hydrogen	H_2	H–H
Hydrogen bromide	HBr	H–Br̈
Chlorine	Cl_2	:C̈l—C̈l:

FIGURE 3.5. Lewis structures of a few molecules.

I must hasten to point out that although it may seem as if we are simply adding electrons to a molecule until the duet or octet rule is satisfied, this is not exactly what is going on. In fact, we have to figure out the total number of valence electrons the molecule is supposed to have by adding up the valence electrons that each atom contributes. In the case of HBr (see Figure 3.5), the hydrogen contributes one valence electron and the bromine contributes seven, giving a total of eight electrons shown in the Lewis structure of HBr. We'll return to this business of keeping track of the total number of electrons in a moment.

You've already seen some examples in Chapters 1 and 2, so you know that most molecules have many more than two atoms and thus their Lewis structures are naturally more complex. We need to consider three situations in order to deal with more complex bonding: molecules with three or more atoms, molecules with multiple bonds, and the concept of formal charges.

Molecules with Three or More Atoms

The case of molecules with three or more atoms introduces a new concern: How are the atoms arranged? This is really the connectivity issue I raised in Chapter 2 and, as you already saw, answering can get tricky if more than a few atoms are involved. (We will return to how we determine the connectivity of larger molecules in Chapter 5.) As a simple example, however, consider the molecule CH_4 (methane, a component of natural gas). Where is the C? On the end or in the middle? Are the Hs in a line, connected to one another?

If you remember our little mnemonic device that 1–2–3–4 bonds are made by the elements H–O–N–C, that helps. Because hydrogen makes only one bond, you cannot have a chain of hydrogen atoms. As soon as you connect one hydrogen to another, you have a complete molecule—the hydrogen molecule H_2—and that is the end of any further bonding. Thus the "H_4" in CH_4 is misleading without the rules of bonding. Conversely, because carbon likes to make four bonds, putting it in the middle of the molecule makes sense. In fact, the formulas of many small molecules are often written in an order that tells you the connectivity. Plenty of exceptions are out there, but generally the atom listed first is central in the structure, unless the molecule is so small that the connectivity is simply the order of the atoms as listed.[10] Applying this guideline, the proper Lewis structure of methane is shown in Figure 3.6.

Note that if we count electrons, the Lewis structure of methane has eight (two electrons in each of the four covalent bonds drawn as lines). This is what we expect; the carbon contributes four valence electrons and the four hydrogens contribute one each. Also shown is the Lewis structure of ammonia, NH_3, used as a fertilizer and in some cleaning solutions (count the electrons in the structure and check against what is expected).

Molecules with Multiple Bonds

A molecule such as HCN (hydrogen cyanide or "cyanide gas") raises not only some connectivity issues but also the issue of multiple bonds. Since HCN is a very simple molecule, we can assume that it is connected in the order written: H–C–N. However, we still need to complete the octet/duets for each atom. With the single bond already drawn between hydrogen and carbon (H–C–N), the duet of hydrogen is satisfied. But carbon and nitrogen both have less than an octet, so they will need additional electrons. Two possible methods can be used to figure out how many additional electrons are needed and where to put them.

$$\begin{array}{cc} \overset{\displaystyle H}{\underset{\displaystyle H}{H-\overset{|}{\underset{|}{C}}-H}} & \overset{\displaystyle \cdot\cdot}{H-\overset{}{\underset{\displaystyle H}{N}}-H} \end{array}$$

FIGURE 3.6. Lewis structures of methane (left) and ammonia.

The first method is to count the total number of valence electrons as we did previously, then distribute them as needed to ensure that all atoms that need an octet have it. Based upon the valence electron configurations (which is reflected in the position in the periodic table), each atom brings electrons to the molecule as follows:

H: 1   C: 4   N: 5

This gives a total of ten valence electrons to the HCN molecule. When we write "H–C–N," the two lines represent covalent bonds containing two electrons each, so a total of six electrons remains to be distributed, and we must do it so that carbon and nitrogen both have an octet. With a little experimentation on scratch paper, you will discover that the only way to satisfy the octet rule *and* follow the rules of bonding (1–2–3–4 ↔ H–O–N–C)[11] is to make a triple bond between carbon and nitrogen and place a lone pair of electrons on the N, as shown in Figure 3.7. Do not let the triple bond bother you; this is perfectly acceptable, as is a double bond, as long as you follow the rules of bonding and the octet rule. Carbon dioxide, CO_2, is another example shown in the figure.

The second method for distributing electrons is more useful once you have had some practice. It is rare that chemists actually count electrons unless they are dealing with a very unusual molecule. Instead, they grow accustomed to seeing the atoms in their typical bonding situations. Figure 2.1 illustrated typical bonding arrangements for carbon. Now you know that carbon makes four bonds because it has four valence electrons available to be shared (which is based upon its electron configuration, which in turn is derived from the periodic table). The bonds can range from four single bonds to various combinations of multiple and single bonds.[12] Nitrogen has three valence electrons waiting to be shared, and a lone pair of electrons. Its typical bonding arrangements are shown in Figure 3.8. A similar analysis for oxygen leads to bonding arrangements with two lone pairs and two covalent bonds; this is also shown in Figure 3.8.

H–C≡N :   : Ö=C=Ö :

FIGURE 3.7. Lewis structures of hydrogen cyanide (left) and carbon dioxide.

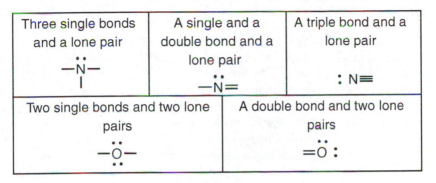

FIGURE 3.8. Typical bonding arrangements for nitrogen and oxygen.

Don't forget that the periodic table tells us that whatever kind of bonding oxygen is willing to undergo, the atoms in the same column in the periodic table will behave similarly. Thus, sulfur (S) will make bonds just as oxygen does, although it is also capable of other bonding arrangements.

Applying the second method to HCN, after writing the connectivity as before (H–C–N) we should add additional bonds between the C and N. In this case, making the bond between C and N triple satisfies C's octet (in general, be sure you don't add any more bonds than the rules of bonding allow). At this point, nitrogen is still not quite up to the octet it requires, so we then add a lone pair to it, giving the same answer as before.

This second method of distributing electrons requires that you connect the atoms first, and then fill in with multiple bonds and finally lone pairs so that each element has a familiar bonding arrangement and thus its octet/duet of electrons. It's a question of whether you want to count electrons every time or do enough examples that the common arrangements become familiar. It takes practice to become comfortable with this method. The more Lewis structures you try, the better you will get and the easier you will ultimately find it to draw molecular structures.

Formal Charge

The last detail of bonding that needs to be addressed is the concept of formal charge. Some atoms that are covalently bonded have a charge on them because they are not sharing their electrons equally. Because some atoms are charged, the entire molecule may be charged (and we would call this an ion). In Figure 3.6, we saw the molecule ammonia, NH_3. Ammonia can react with a proton,[13] H^+, to give a new molecule called the ammonium ion, NH_4^+, as shown in Figure 3.9. The ammonium ion has a charge on it because the lone pair of electrons that was on the NH_3 is now being shared with the hydrogen via a covalent bond. This formal charge, as it is called, resides on the nitrogen atom. Formal charge (FC) is calculated one atom at a time as follows:

$$FC = \text{Valence electrons} - \text{Electrons "owned"}$$

The electrons owned by an atom include all electrons in lone pairs and half of the electrons in any covalent bond to that atom. (Don't confuse this method of counting with the counting method used for the octet rule, which includes *all* electrons surrounding a given atom. *They are different counting methods which are routinely confused.*) So for NH_3 in Figure 3.9, the nitrogen owns the entire lone pair (two electrons) and half of the six electrons in the three covalent bonds, for a total of five electrons. Since nitrogen has five valence electrons, and owns five electrons in this case, it has a formal charge of zero in NH_3.

However, for NH_4^+, the nitrogen no longer completely owns its lone pair (it's being shared in a covalent bond to hydrogen). Instead, this nitrogen owns half of the eight electrons in the four covalent bonds, or four electrons. With five valence electrons, and subtracting the four owned electrons, we reach a formal charge of +1, which we draw next to the nitrogen atom in the Lewis structure.

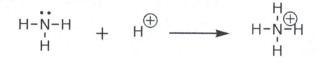

FIGURE 3.9. Ammonia reacting with a proton to create an ammonium ion.

As a final example that embodies all of the issues concerning Lewis structures, let's look at the bicarbonate ion, HCO_3^-. Drawing a proper Lewis structure for this molecule requires determining the connectivity, satisfying the octet rule using multiple bonds and lone pairs (but following the rules of bonding), and determining where the charge is located (since it is an ion, there will be at least one formal charge somewhere in the molecule). An earlier note (you do read them, don't you?) pointed out that hydrogen is sometimes listed first in a formula, but it can never be the central atom because it forms only one bond. In this case the carbon is central, surrounded by the oxygens, and the hydrogen is bonded to one of the oxygens. Figure 3.10, part a, shows the connectivity.

From here, we need to add electrons until we have the correct total, and naturally we must do so following the octet rule (and hopefully keeping in mind common bonding situations so that it goes faster). After adding multiple bonds, we have the structure in Figure 3.10, part b, and then after adding lone pairs we have the structure in Figure 3.10, part c. Finally, we have to check for formal charges. This requires inspecting each atom for an excess or deficiency of electrons as described earlier.[14] The final complete Lewis structure is given in Figure 3.10, part d.

Ionic versus Covalent Bonding

I have presented ionic bonding as the transfer of electrons between two elements, and covalent bonding as the sharing of electrons between two elements. This puts them at opposite extremes because transferring of electrons sounds a lot like *taking* electrons, not sharing them. The share versus transfer extremes are useful simplifications of bonding behavior that help us remember the two types. In reality, however, the majority of bonds have some ionic character *and* some

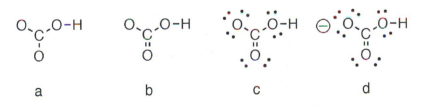

a   b   c   d

FIGURE 3.10. Drawing the Lewis structure of bicarbonate ion.

covalent character. This is because most pairs of elements don't really want to share their electrons equally. It is useful to imagine bonding as a tug-of-war; a really strong element might overcome a weaker element and the so-called sharing might end up as a taking, or transfer. One can cite examples of pure ionic bonds and pure covalent bonds but also many degrees of gray in between; we'll return to this in the next section on molecular properties.

As a final example illustrating both kinds of bonding, let's examine the molecule delphinidin, shown in Figure 3.11. Delphinidin is one of the pigments responsible for the color of blueberries.

In delphinidin, all of the bonds are covalent and every atom has the expected octet or duet. You will note that one of the oxygens has a formal positive charge, making delphinidin as a whole a cation, which could potentially participate in an ionic bond. No anion (a negatively charged atom or molecule) is specified in this case, however, because the anion could be any one of the many anions present in all cells, and in any case the exact identity of the anion is rather irrelevant in a cellular context. Many molecules of medicinal interest in plants have features of both kinds of bonding. Although they are primarily composed of covalent bonds, they sometimes have formal charges on them that will give them, at least in principle, the ability to also participate in ionic bonds. Formal charges also impart certain other properties that we are about to consider.

To summarize this section, remember that ionic and covalent bonding are both driven by the "desires" of the elements to achieve the valence electron configuration of the inert gases. Electron configurations are the underlying, organizing principle of the periodic table, which in turns reminds us of the rules of bonding. Together, this information tells us how to draw the Lewis structures of molecules.

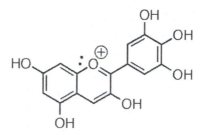

FIGURE 3.11. Delphinidin.

Figure 3.12 summarizes the typical covalent bonding situations of our favorite elements, including those situations involving formal charges.

PREDICTING PROPERTIES
FROM MOLECULAR STRUCTURE

Throughout the preceding discussion of electron configurations and bonding you may well have been thinking, "What's the use of this stuff? Why can't I just use the simple rules of bonding that you gave

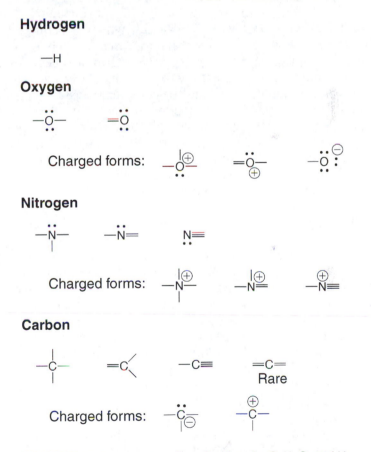

FIGURE 3.12. Common bonding situations for C, N, O, and H.

earlier?" Those darn electrons are fairly important in understanding how drug molecules behave, so we really can't ignore them. We are now ready to talk about molecular shapes and some consequences of molecular shape, and we'll see that an understanding of electrons is critical to these topics.

Molecular Shapes

To understand how a molecule can exert a beneficial or toxic effect on an organism, we must have a clear understanding of its shape.[15] Although thus far we have drawn molecules as two-dimensional objects on two-dimensional paper, they are in most cases three-dimensional. As we will see in more detail in Chapter 6, medicinal molecules interact with what we call a target, which is another, larger molecule that is also three-dimensional (one major group of targets is called the receptors, so I will also use that term at times). Without spoiling the surprise, let me just say for now that the shape of the medicinal molecule and its target must be complementary. Think of how a hand fits in a glove: Many alterations of the glove's design would make the fit of the hand impossible (and some alterations would still allow it). Thus, to understand how a molecule can exert a medicinal effect, we need to understand its shape and some properties that are derived from its shape. Shape is not the only thing we'll need to know, but it's an appropriate starting point.

VSEPR Theory

Fortunately, there is a very simple and powerful theory to help us with the shapes of molecules. It is called VSEPR theory, which stands for valence shell electron pair repulsion theory. You already know what valence shell electrons are; they are the electrons involved in bonding, plus any lone pairs (in other words, the electrons we draw in a Lewis structure). The other part of the theory's name is repulsion, which is simply a reminder that electrons, which are negatively charged, repel one another. A simple, practical statement of the VSEPR theory would be that because electrons repel one another, groups of electrons (either bonding or lone pairs) around a central atom try to get as far away from one another in three-dimensional space as possible. The shape that results depends only upon the number of groups of electrons around the central atom.

The Three Basic Electron Pair Geometries

It is easiest to illustrate the application of VSEPR theory with a simple example. Suppose you have an imaginary atom that we'll call A, which has two other atoms bonded to it and no lone pairs (let's call the other atoms M since they are a mystery, and M is not a symbol for a real element). Thus, A has two bonding pairs of electrons surrounding it. What sort of molecular shape do we get if we let those two pairs of electrons repel each other and move so that they are as far from each other as possible? If you think about this a little, you should conclude that all three atoms will be in a line (see Figure 3.13). If either M atom deviates from that straight line, the electrons that hold it to A would be getting closer to the other pair of electrons, which would not be a good thing, because the electron pairs repel each other. Thus if M were to wiggle a little, it would quickly be forced back to its original spot. For obvious reasons, chemists call this molecular shape linear, and one sees it when two groups of electrons are present around a central atom. Implicit in the term *linear* is the idea that the bond angle (the angle between the atoms M–A–M) is 180°.

What happens if three groups of electrons are present around a central atom? Imagine another hypothetical molecule, AM_3. With a little more mental gymnastics, you'll find that the shape that gets the three groups of electrons as far from each other as possible is a planar shape with the angles between the atoms of 120° (angle M–A–M = 120°). This shape is described as trigonal planar, and is shown in Figure 3.14, part a. In this case, if any of the M atoms moves in the plane of the molecule (the plane of the paper as drawn) by wiggling back and forth, it gets closer to another bonding pair of electrons. The same is true if an M atom moves out of the plane of the molecule by moving closer or further from our viewpoint. The outcome is the same if the formula of the molecule is AM_2 and there is a lone pair of electrons on A, as in Figure 3.14, part b. This is because the lone pair of elec-

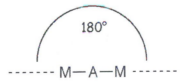

FIGURE 3.13. Linear shape.

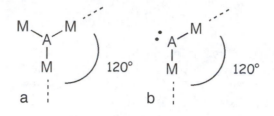

FIGURE 3.14. Trigonal planar shape.

trons has the same effect as a bonded pair of electrons. All we are interested in is how many *groups* of electrons are around a central atom. Whether they are involved in a bond or they are a lone pair owned entirely by the central atom does not matter for the purpose of determining shape. Notice that I have been using the phrase *groups of electrons* rather than *pairs of electrons.* This is because a multiply bonded atom, which would involve more than two electrons, is treated as a single group or object for VSEPR purposes. We will see this illustrated very shortly.

What if we continue to build up our hypothetical molecule and add a fourth group of electrons, making AM_4? In this case we are finally forced to truly think in three dimensions, and most people cannot reach an answer solely by picturing the problem in the mind's eye. A more rigorous derivation tells us that the shape which results is a tetrahedron, where the M atoms are at the corners of the tetrahedron and the A atom is in the center of the tetrahedron. This is shown in Figure 3.15. With some math, one can determine that all the angles in this shape are 109.5°. Fortunately, for the molecules we are interested in we need not go beyond four pairs of electrons around the central atoms. Figure 3.16 provides some examples of molecules where there is only a single central atom. By the way, there is nothing special about having the same kinds of atoms surrounding the central atom; we just do so to keep it simple. The overall shape of CH_3Cl and CH_4 are the same, for example.

An important concept to grasp is that if you know any one piece of information about the shape of a molecule, you automatically know the others, because they are all equal expressions. For example, if someone tells you that the bond angles in a molecule are 120°, you automatically know that three groups are present around the central

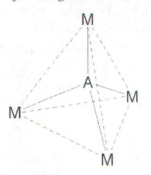

FIGURE 3.15. Tetrahedral shape.

CO_2 (linear)	$\overset{\cdot\cdot}{\underset{\cdot\cdot}{O}}=C=\overset{\cdot\cdot}{\underset{\cdot\cdot}{O}}$
BF_3 (trigonal planar)	$\overset{\cdot\cdot}{\underset{\cdot\cdot}{F}}\diagdown_{B}\diagup\overset{\cdot\cdot}{\underset{\cdot\cdot}{F}}$ $\overset{\mid}{\underset{\cdot\cdot}{\overset{\cdot\cdot}{F}}}$
CH_4 (tetrahedral)	$\overset{H}{\underset{H}{H-\overset{\mid}{\underset{\mid}{C}}-H}}$

FIGURE 3.16. Molecular shape examples.

atom. Similarly, if an atom is referred to as tetrahedral, you instantly know that the bond angles are 109.5°. The important results of VSEPR theory are collected in Table 3.4, which shows these relationships.

Application of VSEPR to Small Molecules

If VSEPR theory is to be really useful, we need to be able to apply it to much larger molecules than we have used as examples. However, because the theory really only considers one atom and the electrons immediately around it at a time, we have to be careful if we are to accurately deal with larger molecules. As further examples, let's continue looking at hydrocarbons. Previously I indicated that methane

TABLE 3.4. Summary of VSEPR theory.

Name	Groups around the central atom	Bond angles
Linear	2	180°
Trigonal planar	3	120°
Tetrahedral	4	109.5°

(CH_4, a saturated hydrocarbon) has a tetrahedral shape. What about the simplest alkene with formula $CH_2=CH_2$ (this is called ethene)? First of all, realize that from the formula and from the rules of bonding the connectivity must be as shown in Figure 3.17, part a.

What about the shape? If we focus on the carbon atoms, each of them is bonded to three groups of electrons: to two hydrogen atoms by single bonds, and to the other carbon atom by a double bond. In terms of VSEPR theory, we should treat these as three groups around a central atom, and thus the shape *in the vicinity* of each carbon atom is trigonal planar. However, because some of the atoms in one trigonal plane overlap or are shared with atoms in the other trigonal plane, the entire molecule is planar, as shown in Figure 3.17, part b.

If we turn now to the simplest alkyne, ethyne or HCCH, we see that each carbon atom with its two neighbors should be linear. Since the three atoms that define the line through one end of the molecule, H–C–C, overlap with the three atoms defining a line on the other end of the molecule, C–C–H, the net result is that all four atoms lie on a line, and the molecule as a whole is linear (see Figure 3.18)

We can make a reasonable guess about the shape of any molecule *as long as we can clearly visualize it as being built up from the three basic shapes* (linear, trigonal planar, and tetrahedral). At some point, however, the molecule becomes too large or other complications set in that make this impractical, but the method works well for many molecules. The next few paragraphs provide more examples to illustrate this method. As we do so, we also have an opportunity to practice our Lewis structures and enhance our knowledge a bit.

Formaldehyde is the simplest aldehyde and has the formula H_2CO; some people write it as CH_2O. Its Lewis structure is shown in Figure 3.19, and you can see that the central carbon atom has three groups of electrons around it. Therefore, the entire molecule is planar, and the carbon atom has a trigonal planar shape. Water (H_2O) is obviously a

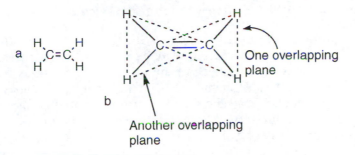

One overlapping plane

Another overlapping plane

FIGURE 3.17. The geometry of ethene. All the atoms lie in the same plane, which is composed of two overlapping planes.

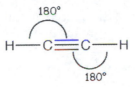

FIGURE 3.18. The geometry of ethyne. All atoms line up.

FIGURE 3.19. Lewis structures of formaldehyde (left) and water.

molecule critical to human life. What is its shape? The Lewis structure in Figure 3.19 shows four pairs of electrons around the central oxygen atom, so we would predict a tetrahedral geometry and a bond angle of 109.5°. Some people refer to water as having a "bent" shape. When they do so, they are thinking only of the atoms, and not of the whole molecule including the lone pairs of electrons. While bent may be an accurate description, it doesn't help us determine the bond angle. Ammonia (NH_3) and methane (CH_4) are other molecules that have a tetrahedral arrangement of groups of electrons (refer back to Figure 3.6).

Application of VSEPR Theory to Larger Molecules

Let's jump right in and try to apply VSEPR theory to determine the shape of a much larger molecule of medicinal interest. As stated earlier, we can estimate the shape of any molecule as long as we can clearly visualize it as being built up from the three basic shapes. This method does not work all the time because the combinations of the basic shapes are limitless. On the other hand, some molecules are built up of primarily one or two basic shapes, and we can get a good feel for the overall molecular shape. An example is hypericin which we saw plenty of in Chapters 1 and 2.

If you study hypericin (in Figure 1.1) in light of what you now know about molecular geometries, you'll see that almost the entire molecule is composed of interlocking groups of trigonal planar carbons (28 of them). Around the perimeter of the molecule are some alcohol groups and two –CH_3 groups that have tetrahedral geometries. Overall, however, if you took a bird's-eye view of hypericin, it would appear planar with just a few hydrogen atoms out of the plane around the edges.

As a second example, consider the molecule thiarubrine A,[16] found in the African plant genus *Aspilia,* which is eaten by chimpanzees to treat intestinal parasites (Figure 3.20).[17] By looking at the ge-

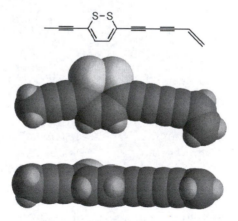

FIGURE 3.20. Thiarubrine A. Top: Lewis structure. Bottom: space-filling views from two perspectives. Atoms are typically colored as follows: carbon—gray; hydrogen—cyan; nitrogen—dark blue; oxygen—red; sulfur—yellow; phosphorous—magenta. See corresponding figure in the color plate section.

ometries of the individual atoms and at how they are connected together, one could describe the shape of this molecule as a nearly flat ring with two rods sticking out from it. Even though the two sulfur atoms are tetrahedral, the lone pairs attached to them don't greatly affect the overall shape of the ring. Because the rest of the ring consists of four trigonal planar carbon atoms, the overall result is a flat ring. The side chains are built from linear carbons (except at the very end of one chain, where they are trigonal planar), so the overall effect is that of a long rod. The figure shows two views of thiarubrine A in space-filling style, which confirm our prediction.

Molecular Flexibility

As we have seen, most smaller molecules have a definite shape. Some special cases of larger molecules have predictable shapes as well. However, as molecules get larger, sooner or later they also become flexible, and this means *they can have multiple shapes* . It is important to have an appreciation of this phenomenon because some of these shapes may fit receptors or targets, and others may not. This means that some shapes of a molecule may have biological activity, and other shapes of the same molecule may not. We will see in Chapter 7 how the flexiblity of certain molecules allows them to mimic the shape of the hallucinogen LSD, and how compounds found in ginkgo can flex to masquerade as naturally occuring molecules and reduce excessive blood clotting.

The flexibility I am speaking of comes about from rotation around single bonds between two carbon atoms.[18] Ethane, CH_3CH_3, provides a simple illustration of the effect of the rotation (see Figure 3.21). If you study these structures, you can see that they have the same connectivity, but they differ in shape because the rear carbon has been rotated relative to the front carbon. Chemists have devel-

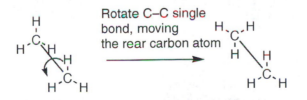

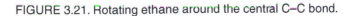

FIGURE 3.21. Rotating ethane around the central C–C bond.

oped another way to view these shapes: a Newman projection. In a Newman projection, one views the molecule looking down or along a C–C bond, much as if one was looking down a narrow tube. In a Newman projection, one carbon atom is near you, and is represented by the intersection of the three lines leading to three bonded atoms. The other carbon is farther away, hidden behind the first carbon atom. We represent the far carbon with a large circle, which again has three bonds leading away from it. It may appear that each carbon has only three bonds; this is because the fourth bond is between the two carbons and viewed end-on (and therefore essentially hidden). Figure 3.22 shows how to relate the two ways of drawing the two unique forms of ethane. In the upper-right Newman projection, the rear carbon is drawn slightly rotated from its true position so that the hydrogens are visible. In reality, the hydrogens on the rear carbon are directly behind the hydrogens of the front carbon and would be hidden ("eclipsed") if the diagram were not skewed a bit.

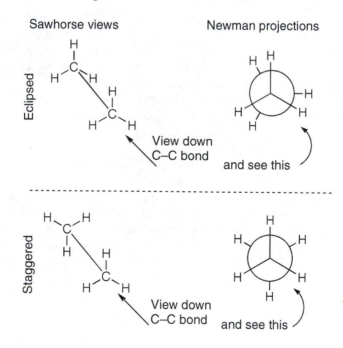

FIGURE 3.22. Views of eclipsed (top) and staggered ethane. Note that the rear atom is drawn slightly offset (rotated) in the eclipsed Newman projection so that the Hs can be seen.

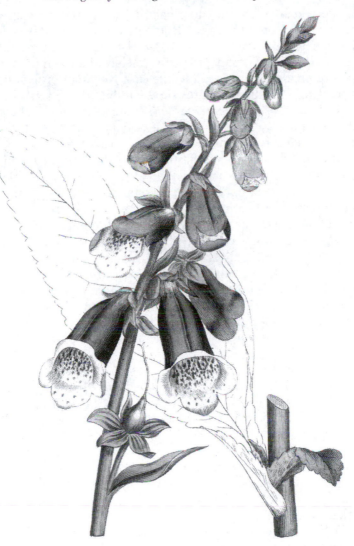

Digitalis purpurea. (*Source:* Woodville, William. *Medical Botany* containing systematic and general descriptions, with pl.s of all the medicinal plants, indigenous and exotic, comprehended in the catalogues of the material medica; as published by the Royal College of Physicians of London and Edinburgh; accompanied with a circumstantial detail of their medicinal effects, and of the diseases in which they have been most successfully employed. London: printed and sold for the author by J. Phillips, 1790, Vol. 1, pl. no. 24.)

If one adds two carbons to ethane to create butane, the possible structures are more numerous. Butane's formula is $CH_3(CH_2)_2CH_3$ which can also be written[19] $CH_3CH_2CH_2CH_3$; we can rotate around three carbon-carbon bonds. If you rotate around the middle carbon-carbon bond and view the molecule in a Newman projection along that bond, you get the structures shown in Figure 3.23. It's important to realize that *these structures are all forms of butane.* In fact, if you could somehow watch one molecule of butane with a video camera, you would see it rotate through all these structures above over a period of time. The individual structures of butane shown in Figure 3.23, which differ by rotation around a carbon-carbon bond, are called conformers or conformations. This is another type of isomerism (we introduced isomerism due to connectivity in Chapter 2). If we continue to add carbons so that we have a long chain of carbons held together by single bonds, it is possible to rotate around each carbon-carbon single bond. This means that many different conformations are possible; a chain of ten carbons would be a very flexible molecule indeed, and would have no particular shape.

On the other hand, when carbons are formed into ring structures, the closing of a floppy chain to form a ring limits the flexibility of the whole molecule. Rings of six saturated carbons turn out to be very common in plant drug molecules, and we should look at them a bit closer. The simplest example is a molecule called cyclohexane. I can't write a condensed formula for it because of the ring, but its two-dimensional structure is shown in Figure 3.24, part a, and several styles of drawing it in perspective are shown in Figure 3.24, part b. Note that the "thick" bond drawing style means that those bonds and atoms are closer to you; this is a way of indicating perspective or three-dimensional shape on two-dimensional paper (compare to Figure 2.7). Cyclohexane has *some* flexibility due to partial rotation around the C–C bonds. The shape cyclohexane prefers to assume is the chair; Figure 3.24, part b shows views of this chair. Why is this called a "chair"? Imagine yourself sitting in it, as indicated in Figure 3.24, part c.

As mentioned, cyclohexane chairs show up frequently in plant molecules. One such example is the molecule digitoxigenin, which has a powerful effect on the heart and can be either a poison or a medicine, depending upon dose. It is one of several structurally related molecules found in the foxglove *Digitalis purpurea* and it contains three interlocking chairs. Examine Figure 3.24, part d, to see these chairs.

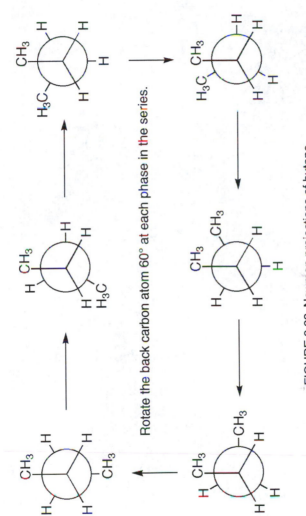

Rotate the back carbon atom 60° at each phase in the series.

FIGURE 3.23. Newman projections of butane.

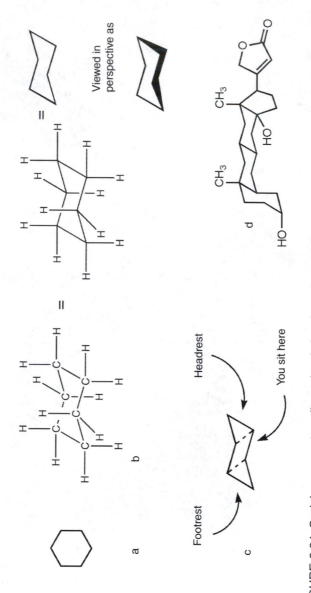

FIGURE 3.24. Cyclohexane. a: two-dimensional view; b: various perspective views; c: the chair; d: digitoxigenin, a molecule with several chairs embedded in the structure.

Occasionally, cyclohexane rings are forced into a different, less-preferred shape called a "boat." One usually sees the boat only when other structural features in a molecule force a ring into the boat form. The well-known antimalarial compound quinine (from the South American genus *Cinchona*) is a good illustration. The boat and quinine are illustrated in Figure 3.25. Both digitoxigenin and quinine are good examples of how chairs and boats, embedded in larger structures, influence the shape of the molecule. In these cases, because more than one ring is present and the rings interlock to some degree, a major portion of the molecule is quite rigid.

The concepts described in these sections can help us estimate the shape of many molecules. The shape (and implicitly size) then determines if a molecule will physically fit into a receptor (the complementary shape concept mentioned earlier). However, just because a molecule fits into a receptor doesn't mean it will cause anything to happen; shape is only about half of the picture. Another part of the picture is polarity—a molecular property that depends upon shape.

Polarity

Polarity is a very important concept in chemistry and pharmacology. Among other things, polarity determines if a molecule will dissolve in water and if it can pass the membrane that surrounds the human brain—two properties that are critical in getting drugs to where

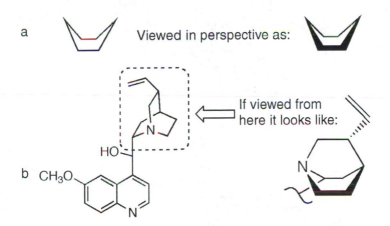

FIGURE 3.25. Cyclohexane boats. a: the boat; b: a boat embedded in quinine.

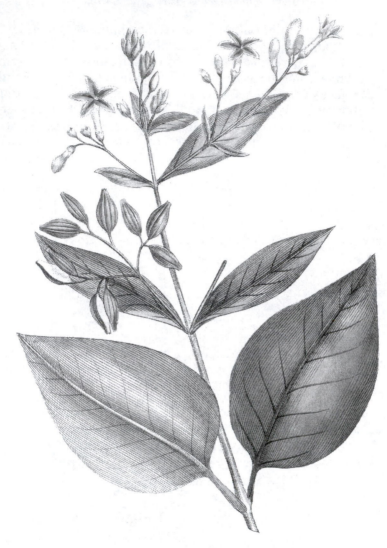

Cinchona major. (*Source:* Woodville, William. *Medical Botany* containing systematic and general descriptions, with pl.s of all the medicinal plants, indigenous and exotic, comprehended in the catalogues of the material medica; as published by the Royal College of Physicians of London and Edinburgh; accompanied with a circumstantial detail of their medicinal effects, and of the diseases in which they have been most successfully employed. London: printed and sold for the author by J. Phillips, 1793, Vol. 3, pl. no. 200.)

they are needed. Polarity also has a number of very practical applications in the laboratory, some of which we will discuss in detail in Chapter 5. For now, we will lay out the basic concepts of polarity.

Polarity refers to the separation of charge in a molecule. Most of the time, but not always, we are not talking about the formal charges previously discussed. Instead, we are dealing with *partial* charges. These partial charges arise because, as mentioned earlier, many covalent bonds do not involve a truly equal sharing of electrons. Some atoms are like bullies or electron hogs, trying to pull the so-called shared electrons toward themselves. Each element has a property called electronegativity, which is a measure of how strongly that atom pulls electrons to itself in a bonding situation. Once again the periodic table provides a way to remember electronegativities—the elements to the right side and at the top of the periodic table have the greatest electronegativity, as seen in Table 3.5.

Thus, fluorine (F) is the most electronegative element, and cesium (Cs) is the least.[20] The elements that interest us most are in the upper right-hand part of the periodic table. Here, for example, are some orders of electronegativity from that region:

$$F > O > N > C$$

$$F > Cl > Br > I$$

We can use the trends in electronegativity to see how they give rise to partial charges, which in turn make polar molecules. For instance, the electrons in the bond in HBr are pulled toward the bromine, because bromine is very electronegative compared to hydrogen. These electrons are not being shared equally. On the other hand, it is still a covalent bond; if the unequal sharing went as far as actually taking electrons we'd be looking at an ionic bond. Chemists illustrate this unequal sharing by using the symbol δ^- next to an atom to indicate that the atom is relatively electron rich. δ^- should be read verbally as a "partial negative charge" (for instance, one could have a –0.3 charge, but we usually don't get down to specific numbers). The symbol δ^+ next to an atom means that the atom is relatively electron poor or deficient, and should be read as a "partial positive charge." This is illustrated in Figure 3.26, part a. As a comparison, we could ask if the H_2 molecule is polar. Because it is composed of two atoms of the same

TABLE 3.5. Electronegativity trends in the periodic table.

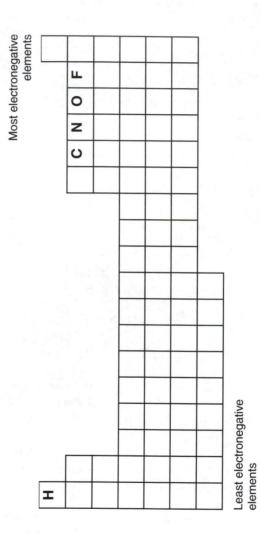

FIGURE 3.26. Polarity of HBr. a: partial charge notation; b: dipole (vector) notation.

element, which by definition have the same electronegativity, the bond in H_2 is truly a pure covalent bond where the electrons are equally shared between the two atoms.

Strictly speaking, we have been discussing bond polarity, which is determined by the *difference* in electronegativity between the two atoms making up the bond. Besides the partial charge symbolism just mentioned, chemists have another way of illustrating the polarity of a bond, which we will use when we move on to larger molecules in just a moment. This other way of illustrating polarity is to draw an arrow from the positive end of the bond toward the negative end of the bond. A cross bar is placed at the positive end of the arrow (see Figure 3.26, part b).[21]

By using this notation and our ability to make predictions about the shapes of molecules, we can extend our analysis of polarity to larger molecules. For example, earlier we determined that ethyne (HCCH), was a linear molecule. Is it polar or nonpolar? To determine this, we need to look at the polarity of each bond and then do a quick summation of the bond dipoles in three dimensions to see what results. I say "quick" because we are only going to estimate the result. We don't have to be perfectly accurate, because we really only need to know if the molecule is obviously polar, obviously nonpolar, or intermediate in polarity. Such estimates are good enough for most applications.

So what about ethyne? Here's how to reason your way to an answer: The carbon-carbon triple bond has no dipole because no difference in electronegativity exists between the two atoms. That leaves two hydrogen-carbon bonds to evaluate. Whatever their dipole is, it is the same for each (see Figure 3.27). Further, because the molecule is linear and symmetrical, the dipoles of the two CH bonds offset each other.[22]

Adding vectors up in three dimensions is not an easy task. Technically, it requires excellent three-dimensional visualization skills and some basic geometry and trigonometry. Chemists don't normally

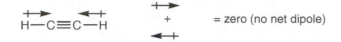

FIGURE 3.27. The polarity of ethyne.

bother with such details, however, because they use shortcuts to make estimates and impress friends.

The first shortcut is that if a molecule has any of the three basic shapes (linear, trigonal planar, or tetrahedral) and it is symmetrically substituted, then it is nonpolar. This statement is true because the various bond dipole vectors will cancel one another out. For instance, CF_4 has very polar bonds and a tetrahedral shape. However, overall it is nonpolar because the vectors add to zero (proving this is tedious, but it's true). Similarly, BCl_3, which is trigonal planar, is nonpolar. This shortcut works for molecules of any size that have various forms of symmetry, but it is usually easier to visualize the symmetry of smaller molecules. For instance, this shortcut can help us decide whether CH_4 or CH_3Cl is more polar. Because CH_4 is symmetrically substituted, we expect it to be totally nonpolar. In contrast, CH_3Cl has a large dipole moment due to the C–Cl bond (compared to the difference in electronegativity between carbon and chlorine, we can safely ignore the CH bond dipoles). The same kind of reasoning would lead us to conclude that benzene (Figure 2.5) is nonpolar due to its symmetry but that hydroxybenzene (or phenol, C_6H_5OH) would have some polarity because the dipoles in the alcohol group are not canceled by any other dipoles.

What about shortcuts to help us estimate the polarity of larger molecules? For very large molecules, there will certainly be far too many bonds to do any kind of vector addition that we would trust, so we need a different method for estimating polarity. The easiest thing to do is to look at the molecule *holistically*. This leads to our second shortcut: If a molecule is mostly hydrocarbon in nature, then we can safely conclude that it is nonpolar (because the difference in electronegativity between C and H is small). On the other hand, if many functional groups with electronegative oxygens and nitrogens are present, and especially if many NH and OH groups are present, the molecule will be polar, unless it is symmetrical. (In large molecules

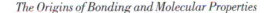
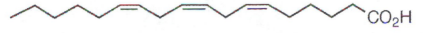

FIGURE 3.28. γ-Linolenic acid.

without symmetry, it is unlikely the bond dipoles are going to cancel each other out.)

The third and final shortcut is to recognize that in some large molecules, some regions may be very nonpolar while other regions may be polar. This observation can be very useful, but it's also good to be able to take a holistic, overall impression of the polarity.[23]

As an example, let's consider γ-linolenic acid, a fatty acid found in plants which is essential to the human diet (Figure 3.28). Is γ-linolenic acid polar or nonpolar? Because the vast majority of the molecule is composed of hydrocarbon, we would have to say it is nonpolar *overall* (shortcut number two). However, one would be wise to note that one end of the molecule is a carboxylic acid which contains two electronegative oxygen atoms. At times it would be useful to think of γ-linolenic acid as a large nonpolar chain with a polar functional group at one end (shortcut number three).

To recap the last part of the chapter, remember that the shape of a molecule depends upon the electron pairs surrounding each individual atom, which is derived from a knowledge of Lewis structures. If we are lucky, we can make an educated guess about the shape of larger molecules, including taking into account the flexibility of single bonds and the presence of any fairly rigid rings. Finally, using the concept of electronegativity and the shortcuts described, we can estimate the polarity of a molecule.

After a technically much lighter tour of important chemical families in the next chapter, we can apply the concepts of bonding and polarity in order to better understand the behavior of medicinally active molecules as described in Chapter 5.

SUGGESTED READING

Strathern, P. (2000). *Mendeleyv's dream:The quest for the elements.* New York: Thomas Dunne Books. A very readable account of science leading up to the development of the periodic table.

Chapter 4

A Structural Lexicon
of Medicinally Important
Chemical Families Found in Plants

Herbs and plants are medical jewels gracing the woods, fields
and lanes which few eyes see, and few minds understand.
Through this want of observation and knowledge the world suffers immense loss.

Linnaeus (1707-1778)

Many times when reading about medicinal plants, you will encounter terms used to describe or name various chemical families.
The purpose of this chapter is to provide you with a brief tour of the
common families of chemicals found in plants, with an emphasis on
those of medicinal interest. For each family a short background is
given, followed by structural examples and any terms commonly
used to describe the families. You can use this section in two ways—
you can skim it to get a general picture of the variety of chemical families that have been found in medicinal plants, or you can simply refer
to it when needed. A few of you might like to read it in detail.

The entries are arranged alphabetically and are divided into two
broad categories: compounds of *primary* metabolism and compounds
of *secondary* metabolism. Primary metabolism refers to the molecules and processes absolutely necessary for life such as energy
sources, genetic material, proteins, and the components of cell membranes. A cell or organism cannot live without each of these categories of molecules in functioning form. Because all organisms have
such molecules, they are generally of little medicinal interest, although I will point out some exceptions.

For example, what would happen if one of the molecules that makes up DNA (deoxyribonucleic acid) were toxic in some way? Because the synthesis and processing of DNA is a central event in all organisms, every organism would need a means of protecting itself from its own toxic material. Given DNA's role in the life of a cell, it seems unlikely that a toxic DNA building block could exist at all. Indeed, none of the building blocks of DNA appear to have any toxic effects on organisms—at least not at the concentrations typically found in cells. This does not rule out, however, the possibility that molecules with broadly similar structure might be of medicinal interest.

Secondary metabolism is much more interesting from the medicinal point of view and will be the main focus of this chapter. Secondary metabolism involves those processes that give rise to molecules which are *not* required for the short-term functioning of an organism. Secondary metabolites are generally considered to be defensive substances; for example, they are often toxic in the animals that eat the plant, such as insects or grazing mammals. Secondary metabolites include, for example, the pigments found in flowers and the volatile molecules used by plants for attracting pollinators. This chapter focuses on examples that have proven medicinally interesting.

COMPOUNDS OF PRIMARY METABOLISM

Carbohydrates

Carbohydrates or sugars have two main functions in plants. First, they act as sources of stored energy. For example, the starch in a potato represents energy stored for new growth. Second, carbohydrates in the form of cellulose provide mechanical strength to plant cells by forming rigid fibers in the cell walls. This wall strength is what allows the so-called higher plants to grow upright in the form of shrubs or trees.

The simplest sugars are called monosaccharides. Glucose is the most important and common, but many others exist. Glucose is shown in Figure 4.1 in some of the different drawing styles you may encounter. Sugars can also be linked together in groups. For example, sucrose is a *di*saccharide found in plants that is composed of the monosaccharides glucose and fructose (see Figure 4.2).

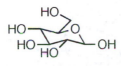 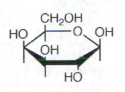 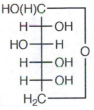

Preferred drawing style   Haworth projection   Fischer projection

FIGURE 4.1. Glucose in various drawing styles.

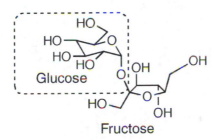

FIGURE 4.2. Sucrose.

Sugars can be linked into longer chains that are called oligosaccha-rides (*oligo-* means "few" or "several") if they have roughly three to ten sugar building blocks. In other cases, the chain may be much longer and may have branches; as a group these molecules are called polysaccharides. Cellulose and starch, mentioned earlier, are good examples. Starch is actually two molecules—amylose and amylopectin. Note that each of these molecules is actually a polymer (long chain) of glucose molecules connected together through different atoms (see Figure 4.3; the arrows in the diagram indicate that the chain continues repeating in a similar manner).

Another class of more complex polysaccharides found in plants are the gums. Examples include alginic acid, carrageenan, and agar found in algae, as well as gum arabic, from the *Acacia* tree. These gums and others similar to them have uses ranging from thickening agents for foods to carriers for medicinal products, and they are water

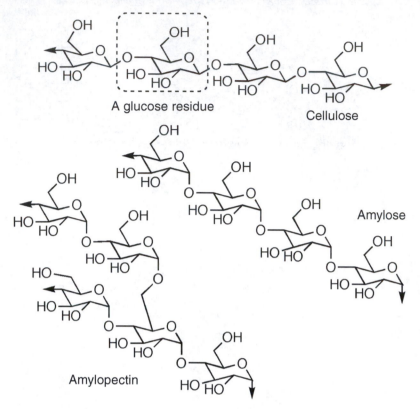

A glucose residue

Cellulose

Amylose

Amylopectin

FIGURE 4.3. Polysaccharides.

soluble (chewing gum is a latex, which is not water soluble). Dietary fiber is also a mixture of several polysaccharides.

For the most part, carbohydrates play a very minor role as medicinal substances. One exception is the North American herb *Echinacea* (purple coneflower), which stimulates the immune system and helps fight off or reduce the severity of an infection. Echinacea's actions appear to be due to several classes of chemicals and, although it is one of the most heavily researched herbs, a complete picture of exactly which molecules are responsible for its beneficial effects has yet to emerge. However, several polysaccharides appear to be important, in part, in the activation of the immune system. Because of their long chains, these molecules are difficult to isolate and identify, and in fact are probably better described as mixtures of closely related isomers. *Plantago major* (common plantain), a European plant naturalized worldwide many centuries ago and used to aid in wound healing, is another plant with biologically active, complex polysaccharides. The aloe plant *Aloe barbadensis)* is another good example of a plant with medicinally active polysaccharides.

Although few mono-, di-, or oligosaccharides have medicinal properties by themselves, they do combine with other medicinally interesting molecules. Such a molecule is referred to as a glycoside. In fact, many medicinally interesting molecules are originally found in nature as glycosides; they are discussed in more detail in their own section later in this chapter.

Lipids

Lipids, also known as fats, are primarily nonpolar hydrocarbon molecules. Some serve as energy sources in plants, particularly in seeds that are rich in cooking oils, such as soybean and corn oil. Certain kinds of lipids are the main components of the membranes that surround the cells in all organisms (membranes are discussed in Chapter 5). The building blocks of lipids are the fatty acids, so called because of their presence in fats. Fatty acids can be saturated or unsaturated. The unsaturated fatty acids include a number that are nutritionally important. Two examples are shown in Figure 4.4.

Generally, fatty acids are not found per se in membranes but are combined with another molecule that links them together. Many different combinations of fatty acids and linking molecules are possible. Representative examples (see Figure 4.5) are the phosphatidylcho-

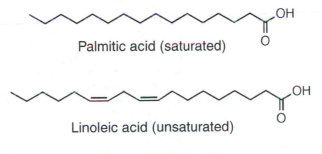

Palmitic acid (saturated)

Linoleic acid (unsaturated)

FIGURE 4.4. Fatty acids.

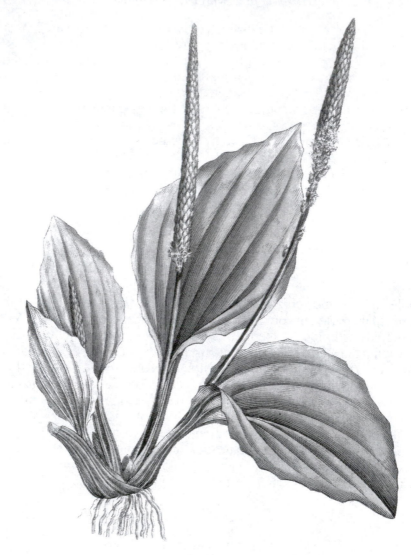

Plantago major. (*Source:* Woodville, William. *Medical Botany* containing systematic and general descriptions, with pl.s of all the medicinal plants, indigenous and exotic, comprehended in the catalogues of the material medica; as published by the Royal College of Physicians of London and Edinburgh; accompanied with a circumstantial detail of their medicinal effects, and of the diseases in which they have been most successfully employed. London: printed and sold for the author by J. Phillips, 1790, Vol. 1, pl. no. 14.)

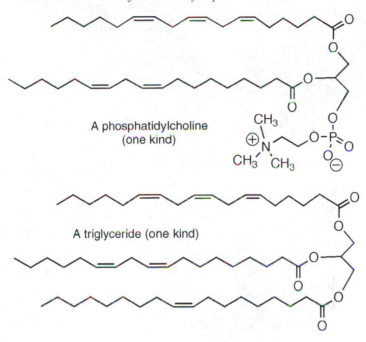

FIGURE 4.5. Examples of lipids from membranes.

lines (also called lecithins), which are composed of two fatty acids linked through the ester group to a polar molecule.

The seed oils (corn, soybean, peanut, etc.) are combinations of three fatty acids connected by an ester bond to the molecule glycerol that yield a triglyceride. Again, many combinations of specific fatty acids are possible. The triglyceride shown in Figure 4.5 is typical of those found in evening primrose oil (from *Oenothera biennis*), which has been used to treat eczema and premenstrual syndrome.

Generally, only a few of the lipids would be considered medicinal.[1] As just mentioned, evening primrose oil has useful healing properties, and several unsaturated fatty acids are needed in the human diet because we cannot synthesize them ourselves (the so-called EFAs—essential fatty acids). The greatest medicinal interest in lipids is not in the lipids themselves but in keeping the lipids structurally intact by ensuring proper levels of antioxidants. This is discussed in detail in Chapter 5.

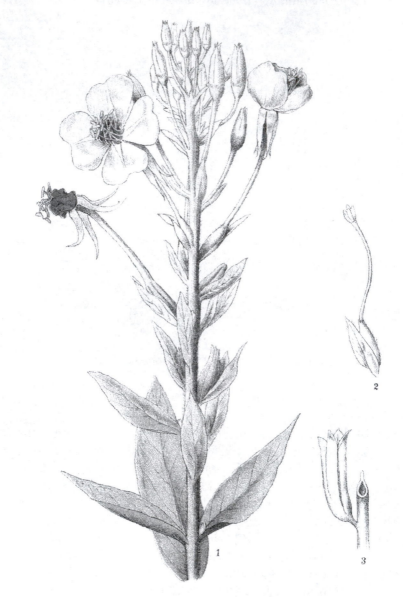

Oenothera biennis. (*Source:* Millspaugh, Charles F. *American Medicinal Plants: An Illustrated and Descriptive Guide to the American Plants Used As Homeopathic Remedies; Their History, Preparation, Chemistry and Physiological Effects.* New York: Boerick & Tafel, 1887. Vol. 1, pl. no. 60.)

Amino Acids and Proteins

Amino acids are, as the name indicates, molecules containing the amine and carboxylic acid functional groups. Their main role in both plants and animals is to be building blocks for proteins, which are polymers (long chains) composed of dozens to hundreds of amino acids. Several examples of amino acids important in proteins are shown in Figure 4.6; a total of 20 are used in construction of proteins, but many more are known that have a variety of other functions. Note that the lower portion of the molecules as drawn in Figure 4.6 are common to all of the amino acids used in proteins; the upper part varies.

Proteins have a variety of functions in the human body. They constitute the structural material of the muscular system (for example, actin in muscles, collagen in skin and ligaments). They serve to transport small molecules (for instance, hemoglobin carries oxygen in the blood). Proteins called enzymes carry out all of the reactions in the body, ranging from the digestion of food to copying DNA, and they serve similar functions in plants.[2] Because proteins can be made from a number of different amino acids, their structures show tremendous variety and complexity (which parallels the variety of functions just described). In the following sections I mention an example of an amino acid derivative and a protein that have a medicinal or toxic effect.

Lectins

Lectins are a complex, difficult-to-study group of molecules that are a special type of glycoprotein, which are protein chains with sugars (the *glyo-* prefix) attached. The word *lectin* comes from the Latin verb "to select," because lectins bind to the sugar residues found on

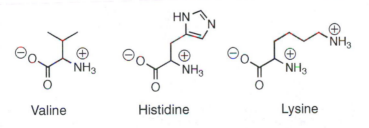

Valine   Histidine   Lysine

FIGURE 4.6. Amino acids typically found in proteins.

the surfaces of cells, often in a very selective manner. Most lectins are found in seeds and are destroyed by cooking. However, a few lectins are not destroyed by cooking or digestive enzymes and are extremely toxic if ingested. For example, the castor bean plant, *Ricinus communis,* contains a lectin called ricin in its seeds which is among the most potent plant toxins known.[3] Ricin has 529 amino acid residues and is composed of two linked chains. One chain binds to the cell-surface sugars, stimulating the cell to bring the ricin molecule inside. Once inside, ricin's other chain interferes with protein synthesis by disabling the protein synthesis apparatus. Other plants containing lectins include mistletoe *(Viscum album)* a parasite of certain trees,

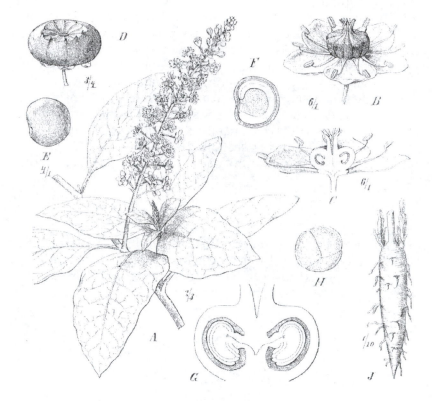

Phytolacca americana. (*Source: Das Pflanzenreich: Regni Vegetabilis Conspectus* heraugegeben von. A. Engler. Leipzig: W. Engelmann, 1909. 39. Heft, IV, 83, Phytolaccaceae, p. 52, fig. 17.)

and pokeweed *Phytolacca americana,* a common roadside inhabitant in the eastern United States. Parts of both plants are toxic but have been used in traditional medicine. The news about lectins is not all bad, however. Portions of highly toxic lectins have been combined with antibodies to recognize cancers cells. The hope is that the antibody will direct the toxic protein chain specifically to the cancer cell, while normal cells will be unaffected.

Because proteins are generally composed of many amino acids, they contain hundreds or even thousands of atoms (over 4,000 are present in ricin). Out of necessity, diagrams intended to help visualize the overall three-dimensional structure of proteins do not show individual atoms very clearly. Two views of ricin are shown in Figure 4.7; the left-hand structure shows the backbone of the protein chain, which is the long chain of carbons and nitrogens to which the remaining atoms are attached. This structure is drawn in ribbon style to emphasize certain features.[4] The right-hand structure is shown in space-filling style to provide a sense of how the atoms pack together to give an overall shape. For clarity, hydrogen atoms are not shown in the right-hand diagram.

MushroomToxins

The deadly mushroom *Amantia phalloides* contains a cyclic peptide (short protein chain) called α-amanitin which is composed of eight amino acid residues. This molecule inhibits the critical enzyme RNA (ribonucleic acid) polymerase II which the body uses to make RNA from DNA. α-Amanitin is one of the most toxic molecules known to humans; consumption of one mushroom cap can readily kill a person by severely damaging the liver (see Figure 4.8).

Cyclotides

Cyclotides are a unique group of cyclic peptides composed of about 30 amino acid residues; they are found largely in species of violets (*Viola* species). They are composed of several rings that assemble to form a knot. The cyclotides have been found to have biological activities ranging from anti-HIV (human immunodeficiency virus) and antimicrobial action to hemolytic (blood-cell bursting) action. In one case, a cyclotide called kalata B1 was discovered based upon reports

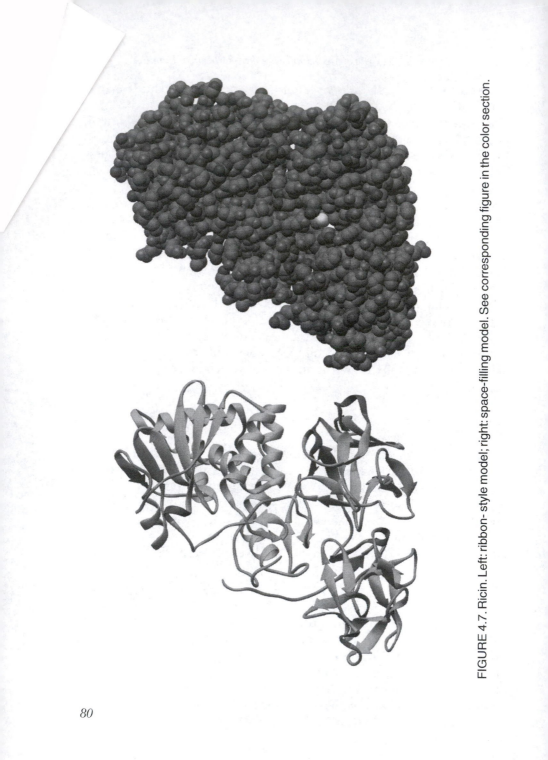

FIGURE 4.7. Ricin. Left: ribbon-style model; right: space-filling model. See corresponding figure in the color section.

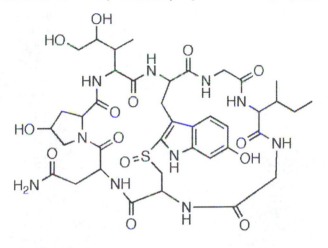

FIGURE 4.8. α-Amanitin.

of the Lulua tribe of Africa, which uses *Oldenlandia affinis* as a child-birth stimulant. Because of their knotted structure, the cyclotides are difficult to illustrate. I mention them because, along with the mushroom toxins, they represent one of the few natural protein or peptide products from plants with medicinal properties.

Nucleic Acids

The nucleic acids DNA and RNA are the genetic material of cells. They are composed of three building blocks: a base, a sugar, and phosphate. There are five bases: adenine (A), thymine (T; found only in DNA), guanine (G), cytosine (C), and uracil (U; found only in RNA). There are two sugars: deoxyribose in DNA and ribose in RNA. These building blocks are assembled into long chains or polymers; the sequence of bases along the chain composes what is commonly called the genetic code. Two long strands of DNA coil together to form the famous double helix; the structure of RNA is more complex and is not considered here. The issues mentioned earlier with visualizing the structures of proteins also arise with visualizing DNA. For comparison, a ball-and-stick view and a space-filling view of a section of DNA containing 12 base pairs are shown in Figure 4.9.

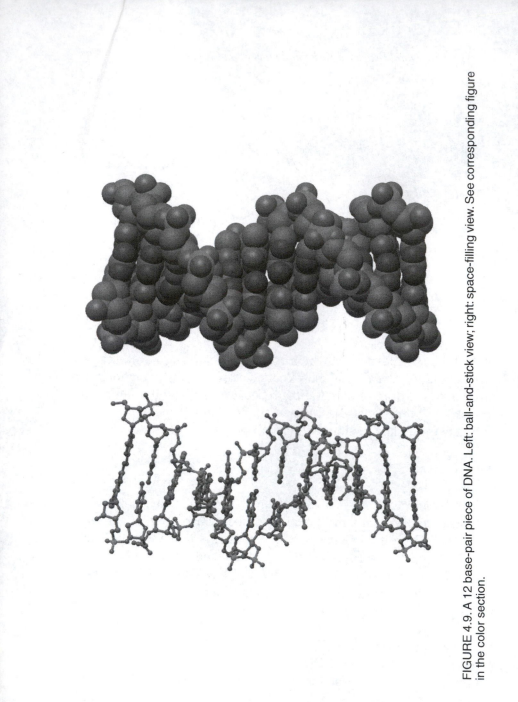

FIGURE 4.9. A 12 base-pair piece of DNA. Left: ball-and-stick view; right: space-filling view. See corresponding figure in the color section.

Relatively few naturally occurring drugs are structurally related to nucleic acids. Caffeine, the morning friend to so many, is an important example. Figure 4.10 shows the structure of caffeine with the base guanine found in DNA and RNA for comparison.

SECONDARY METABOLITES

Alkaloids

Alkaloids are the second largest, most diverse, and most medicinally important group of secondary metabolites, with more than 10,000 structures known.[5] Because of their structural diversity, it is difficult to define them in simple terms. A good working definition for most purposes is that they are molecules which have a nitrogen atom in a ring and which are found in plants. Many people include in the definition that they act as bases,[6] but a number of alkaloids are neutral in their behavior. Sometimes the way a plant makes the molecule (its biosynthesis) is used to classify it as an alkaloid. However, this does not serve very well as a general definition because in some cases the origins are not known, and in any case one has to be a specialist to use this definition. Historically, alkaloids were also recognized as being bitter, but this isn't a useful definition unless you have samples and plan to taste them (quite likely at some risk). A few molecules that are not alkaloids would be inadvertently included by using our simple definition, but for most purposes, including ours, this is inconsequential.

The acid-base behavior exhibited by most alkaloids is important in understanding their bioavailability, which is how well they are ab-

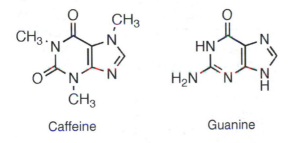

Caffeine   Guanine

FIGURE 4.10. Molecules related to nucleic acids.

sorbed into the bloodstream and get to the site of action (this topic is addressed more fully in Chapter 6; see Figure 6.4). At the pH of plant cells (7.4-7.6), in human blood, and in the highly acidic environment of the human stomach, the nitrogen atom(s) of most alkaloids will bear an extra hydrogen atom and thus carry a positive charge (we say the nitrogen atom is protonated). This makes the molecule polar and readily water soluble (refer to the concepts presented in Chapter 3). The unprotonated form, which is generally what is illustrated in books (including the structures in this chapter), is much less polar and seldom water soluble. These differences can have a dramatic effect on bioavailability and thus the suitability of a molecule for clinical use. Alkaloids for medicinal use are typically provided in the protonated form so that they will dissolve readily in the bloodstream. This behavior is also discussed in more detail in this chapter under the heading Tropane Ring System, using cocaine as an example.

The names of alkaloids are nearly as diverse as their structures. Three main methods of naming are used. One method is to refer to a group of related alkaloids by the common chemical name of one of them that is well-known. For instance, one might use the term *morphine alkaloids* to refer to compounds structurally related to morphine, which is a specific compound from the opium poppy. Another method of naming is to employ the Latin genus or family name of the plant from which a group of alkaloids were originally isolated. The term *Lobelia alkaloids* would refer to the alkaloids found in the genus *Lobelia*. Most of these alkaloids contain a saturated six-membered ring with one nitrogen in it, called a piperidine ring. This illustrates the third common method of naming alkaloids—using the chemical name of the nitrogenous (nitrogen-containing) ring as a descriptor. It would be accurate to say that most *Lobelia* alkaloids are also piperidine alkaloids, but not all piperidine alkaloids are *Lobelia* alkaloids. The only problem with using the ring as the source of the name is that some of the more complex alkaloids contain several nitrogen atoms and multiple rings. A question then arises as to which ring should be used for the name. Usually the choice is a historical one.

The structural lexicon of alkaloids below is organized using this latter method: the chemical name of the nitrogenous ring. I will illustrate the range of structures known by showing the basic ring system and then one or more examples of a particular alkaloid possessing that ring system. I also give a brief background on each example. This

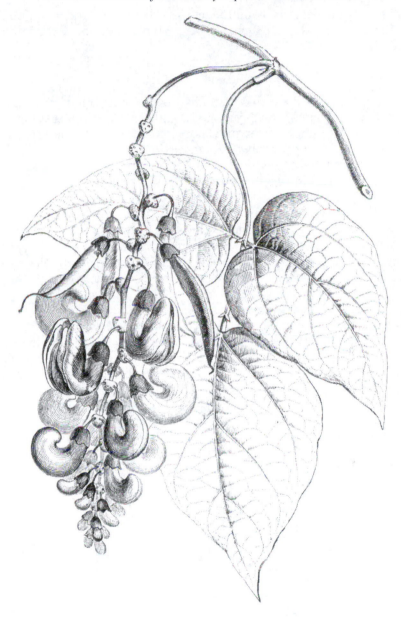

Physostigma venenosum. (*Source:* Baillon, H. *Traite de Botanique Medicale* phanerogamique. Paris: Librarie Hachette, 1884, p. 630, fig. 2191.)

tour will by no means be comprehensive—there is just too much variety in the alkaloids to see them all, so we'll focus on some of notable medicinal interest.

Indole Ring System

Alkaloids based on the indole ring system represent the largest and most diverse group within the alkaloids and contain the most structurally complex examples known. A large number of this group are important either therapeutically or as toxins.

Physostigmine (see Figure 4.11) is obtained from the seeds of the Calabar bean *(Physostigma venenosum),* which historically has been used as an ordeal poison among certain African cultural groups. An ordeal poison served as a trial of sorts. An accused person was made to eat the beans. If he or she survived (usually because the toxic compounds were vomited up), this was taken as evidence of innocence, and if not . . . well, you get the idea. We now know that physostigmine acts on the central nervous system. For many years, it was used clinically for glaucoma, but it has since been replaced by synthetic derivatives.

Another important indole alkaloid is strychnine, a very potent poison isolated from the seeds of nux vomica *(Strychnos nux-vomica),* which is commonly used as rat poison. Reserpine is found in the Indian plant *Rauwolfia serpentina* and was one of the first effective drugs for lowering blood pressure. The psychoactive substance LSD (lysergic acid diethylamide) is also an indole alkaloid; its structure can be found in Figure 7.5. As a final example illustrating the pinnacle of complexity in this group, I offer the structure of vincristine. Isolated from the Madagascan periwinkle (*Catharanthus* or *Vinca roseus*) which is often used as an ornamental bedding plant, vincristine has powerful anticancer activity. These more complex indole alkaloids are shown in Figure 4.12.

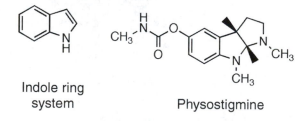

Indole ring
system

Physostigmine

FIGURE 4.11. The indole ring system and a simple indole alkaloid.

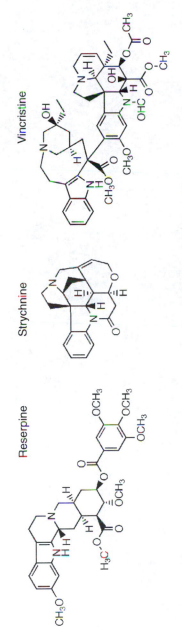

Reserpine

Strychnine

Vincristine

FIGURE 4.12. Structurally complex indole alkaloids.

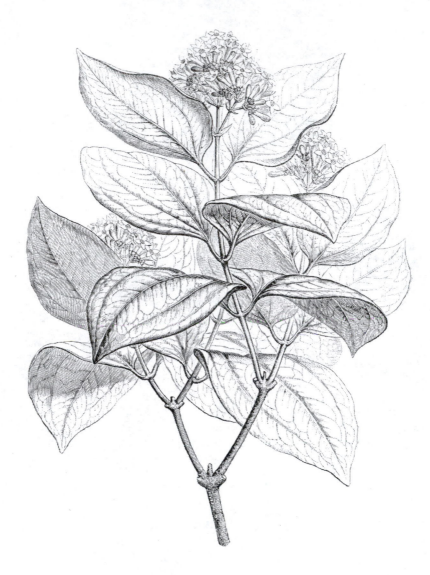

Strychnos nux-vomica. (*Source:* Baillon, H. *Traite de Botanique Medicale phanerogamique.* Paris: Librarie Hachette, 1884, p. 1212, fig. 3126.)

IsoquinolineRingSytem

Alkaloids containing the isoquinoline ring system are probably the second most abundant and diverse family of alkaloids known. Many are of exceptional medical importance. Curare, for example, is the name for a mixture of alkaloids used as a traditional hunting poison in South America. The molecules in curare act by blocking nerve signals where they enter the muscle. The result is that an animal shot with a curare-tipped arrow becomes paralyzed and falls to the ground where it can be captured readily. The flesh is safe to consume because the curare is destroyed by the digestive process. Compounds isolated from curare have been used in surgery as muscle relaxants and anesthetics for some time, although synthetic derivatives based on the original structures are now preferred. Tubocurarine (see Figure 4.13) is an important component of curare.

The bloodroot plant *(Sanguinaria canadensis)* common in eastern North American forests in the spring, exudes a red latex when broken. This latex contains sanguinarine, which has antimicrobial and antifungal properties.[7] It is also used in toothpastes because it binds to dental plaque and inhibits bacterial growth. Numerous other medically important examples of isoquinoline alkaloids can be found in the opium poppy *(Papaver somniferum)* Morphine is a classic example and was the first alkaloid to be isolated in pure form, in 1805. These structures are shown in Figure 4.14.

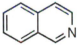

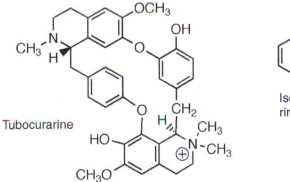

Isoquinoline
ring system

Tubocurarine

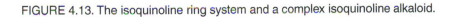

FIGURE 4.13. The isoquinoline ring system and a complex isoquinoline alkaloid.

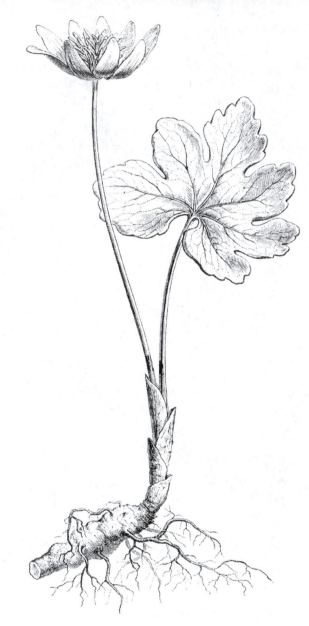

Sanguinaria canadensis. (*Source:* Baillon, H. *Traite de Botanique Medicale phanerogamique.* Paris: Librarie Hachette, 1884, p. 735, fig. 2323.)

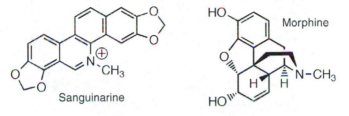

FIGURE 4.14. Further examples of isoquinoline alkaloids.

Pyridine, Piperidine, and Pyrrolidine Ring Systems

The pyridine ring system and its saturated relative, piperidine, are frequently seen in alkaloids. A good example is lobeline, which is a bronchodilating compound found in Indian tobacco *(Lobelia inflata)*. Other interesting examples are nicotine from tobacco (note that the smaller ring is from the pyrrolidine ring system) and piperine, responsible for the pungent taste of black pepper *(Piper nigrum)*. Figure 4.15 illustrates these compounds.

Pyrrolizidine Ring System

Many pyrrolizidine alkaloids are found in the ragworts (genus *Senecio*) where they pose problems for grazing animals (see Figure 4.16). The alkaloids are not directly toxic, but after they are metabolized in an animal's liver, they are converted to a reactive species which then irreversibly damages the liver. Cases of human poisoning and death from the use of herbal products contaminated with plants containing pyrrolizidine alkaloids have been recorded in the United States. Comfrey *(Symphytum officinale)* is an herb whose leaves are frequently used to treat skin conditions. Although one occasionally reads that it can be taken internally, this is an extremely bad idea due to the presence of the pyrrolizidine alkaloid symphytine.[8]

Quinoline Ring System

This alkaloid family has relatively few representatives. Quinine, the antimalarial compound from *Cinchona* species that was so important during World War II, is probably the best known example (see Figure 4.17).

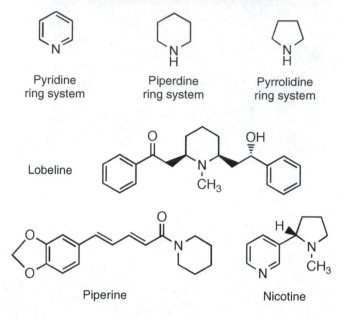

Pyridine
ring system

Piperdine
ring system

Pyrrolidine
ring system

Lobeline

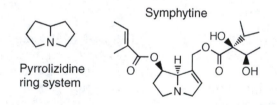

Piperine

Nicotine

FIGURE 4.15. Pyridine, piperidine, and pyrrolidine alkaloids.

Symphytine

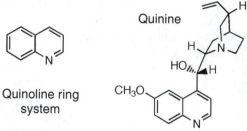

Pyrrolizidine
ring system

FIGURE 4.16. Pyrrolizidine alkaloids.

Quinine

Quinoline ring
system

FIGURE 4.17. Quinoline alkaloids.

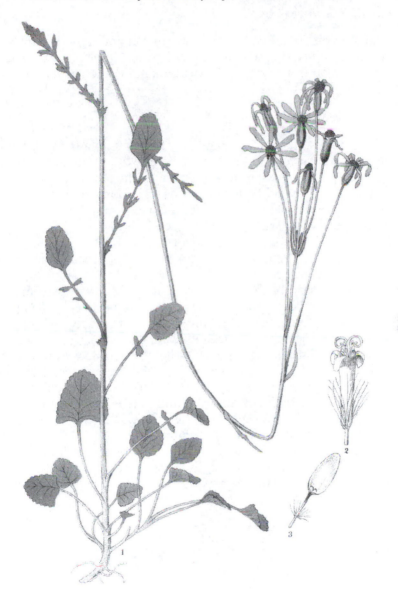

Senecio aureus. (*Source:* Millspaugh, Charles F. *American Medicinal Plants: An Illustrated and Descriptive Guide to the American Plants Used As Homeopathic Remedies; Their History, Preparation, Chemistry and Physiological Effects.* New York: Boerick & Tafel, 1887. Vol. 1, pl. no. 91.)

Quinolizidine Ring System

Quinolizidine alkaloids are frequent in, but not limited to, the bean or legume family (Fabaceae). The beautiful lupines (*Lupinus* spp.) contain numerous toxic quinolizidine alkaloids such as lupinine and anagyrine (see Figure 4.18).

Tropane Ring System

The tropane alkaloids are relatively few in number but very important medically. Several of them are clinically important drugs that act on the central nervous system. Others have a history of poisoning, either accidental or deliberate. Perhaps the most familiar example would be the drug of abuse, cocaine, isolated from the coca plant of South America (*Erythroxylon coca;*   see Figure 4.19). As a drug of abuse, it is usually either snorted or smoked.[9] The snorted form, which found the earliest abuse, is cocaine hydrochloride, which means that the nitrogen atom is protonated and its positive charge is offset by a negatively charged chloride ion. This form is readily absorbed through the mucous membranes of the nose. For a long time this was the preferred form of taking the drug, until people discovered you could also "freebase" cocaine to create "crack" or "rock," and then smoke it. Freebasing means treating the hydrochloride salt with a basic substance to deprotonate the nitrogen, leaving the "free base" or just plain cocaine (see Figure 4.19).[10] This form of cocaine can be smoked, which volatilizes the drug and gets it into the lung tissue where it can be absorbed slightly faster. (Cocaine hydrochloride cannot be smoked because the heat decomposes the drug.) Preparing the freebase in your home has some dangers associated with it, and drug dealers, who are generally very savvy marketers, were quick to address this concern—by the early 1980s crack cocaine was readily available on the street.

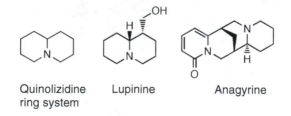

Quinolizidine   Lupinine   Anagyrine
ring system

FIGURE 4.18. Quinolizidine alkaloids.

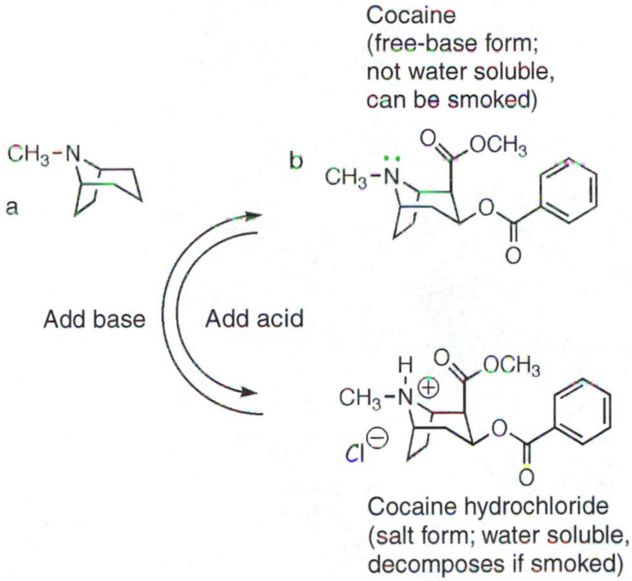

FIGURE 4.19. Tropane alkaloids. a: tropane ring system; b: acid-base behavior of cocaine.

Allium (Garlic) Compounds

The genus *Allium* contains two important culinary herbs, garlic and onion, as well as their close relatives such as chives, shallots, and leeks. These plants have a long history of use in folk medicine and are rich in medicinally important sulfur-containing compounds derived from the amino acid cysteine. The chemistry behind these compounds and their actions is very complex, and for many years it was misunderstood because the compounds are so delicate that their structures changed under the conditions initially used to isolate them. In addition, the compounds present in the intact vegetables have proven to be different from the compounds present in the chopped vegetables, and still other compounds are formed during cooking. Fortunately, each set of compounds confers useful, if different, medicinal properties. With the advent of newer and gentler analytical methods, we now have a very comprehensive understanding of this interesting set of molecules.

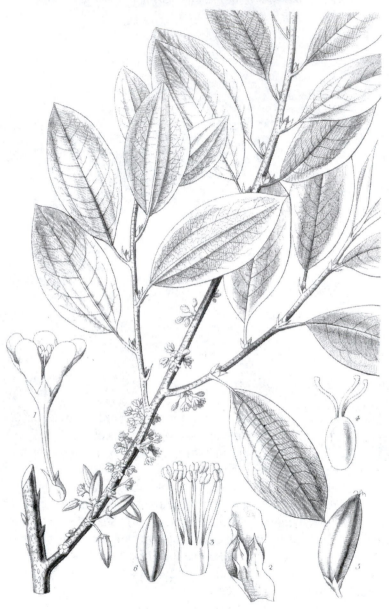

Erythroxylon coca. (*Source: Companion to the Botanical Magazine.* London. Printed by E. Conchman for the proprietor, S. Curtis, 1836. Vol. 2, pl. no. 21.)

Although a wide variety of molecules are found in these plants, I illustrate only a couple of examples here. Allicin (see Figure 4.20), produced by enzyme action when garlic is cut or crushed, has potent antimicrobial and antifungal properties, as well as the ability to inhibit platelet aggregation.[11] Ajoene, also from garlic, has many of the same properties and also inhibits one of the enzymes responsible for fat digestion. This latter property is believed to be responsible for the lowered blood lipid levels seen in people who regularly consume garlic. A compound found in onion, cepaene, shows antiasthma properties by interfering with several of the steps leading to inflammation and bronchoconstriction. The sulfur-sulfur bonds in these unusual compounds are an important part of how they function on a molecular level.

Anthocyanidins and Flavonoids

Anthocyanidins and flavonoids are a very large group of compounds whose primary role in plants is to act as pigments. In humans, they exhibit many desirable medicinal activities; it appears that most of the observed effects are due to their antioxidant properties (discussed in detail in Chapter 5). The basic ring structure common to all members of the group is shown in Figure 4.21. The R group is either H or OH, and the middle ring can have additional alcohols, ketones, and/or double bonds, depending upon the particular subfamily. The alcohol groups are frequently bound to sugars as glycosides.[12]

Preparations of the maidenhair or ginkgo tree *(Ginkgo biloba)* are one of the more popular herbal supplements worldwide. Extracts of this ancient Asian tree protect the tiny capillaries of the brain, leading

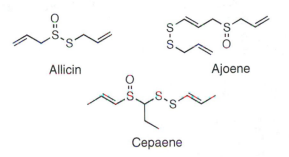

Allicin   Ajoene

Cepaene

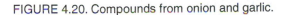

FIGURE 4.20. Compounds from onion and garlic.

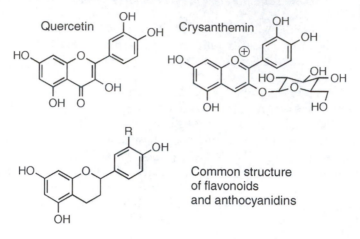

FIGURE 4.21. Flavonoids and anthocyanidins.

to improved cognitive function and protection against stroke. Flavonoid compounds, along with other compounds, are responsible for this activity (see Chapter 7 for a more detailed discussion of ginkgo's actions). An example of one of the vascular-protective flavonoids is quercetin, which is also found in numerous other plants (see Figure 4.21). The chief structural difference between flavonoids and anthocyanidins (and anthocyanins) is that in the latter, the oxygen in the middle ring bears a positive charge. The medicinal activity of the anthocyanidins and anthocyanins appears to be similar to the flavonoids. Cyanin is one of the blue pigments found in blueberries (*Vaccinium mytillus*.) Delphinidin, discussed in Chapter 3, is another example of an anthocyanidin (see Figure 3.11). Note that proanthocyanins are a type of tannin and are discussed under that heading.

Coumarins

Simple Coumarins

Coumarins are a widely distributed group of molecules with a variety of medicinal uses. Coumarin, a compound in its own right, shows the basic ring structure characteristic of the group. Aesculin, a glycoside isolated from the bark of the common horse chestnut (*Aesculus hippocastanum),* acts as a vascular protective agent. It appears to "toughen up" the capillaries, and the plant has been recommended for swelling of the lower legs, hemorrhoids, and varicose veins.[13] Calanolide A, isolated from the fruit and twigs of *Calophyllum lanigerum,* is a coumarin that inhibits the activity of the reverse transcriptase enzyme which is an important molecule in the HIV virus. These structures are shown in Figure 4.22.

Furanocoumarins

The furanocoumarins are photoreactive relatives of coumarins. These molecules can produce photodermatitis when the plant oils, containing furanocoumarins, get on the skin. Subsequent exposure to sunlight causes irritation and sometimes blisters. A long-lasting hyperpigmentation may also result. This photosensitizing behavior has been put to use as a means of treating psoriasis and other skin disorders. Species such as angelica (*Angelica* spp.) and wild parsnip *(Pastinaca sativa)* are typical examples of plants containing furanocoumarins. Furanocoumarins such as bergapten can react with thymines found in DNA to cause "lesions" which distort the structure of the DNA by cross-linking it. This is probably responsible for the dermatitis, although it has not been proven, and certainly explains the carcinogenic properties of these molecules. Figure 4.23 illustrates bergapten reacting with DNA.

Cyanogenic Glycosides

An important group of molecules derived from amino acids are the cyanogenic glycosides. Glycosides are molecules combined with

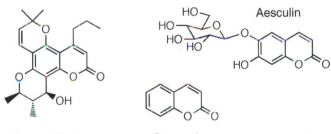

Calanolide A   Coumarin

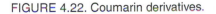

FIGURE 4.22. Coumarin derivatives.

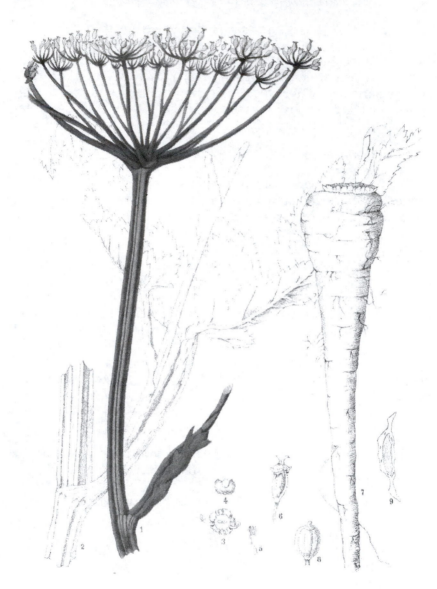

Pastinaca sativa. (*Source:* Millspaugh, Charles F. *American Medicinal Plants: An Illustrated and Descriptive Guide to the American Plants Used As Homeopathic Remedies; Their History, Preparation, Chemistry and Physiological Effects.* New York: Boerick & Tafel, 1887. Vol. 1, pl. no. 63.)

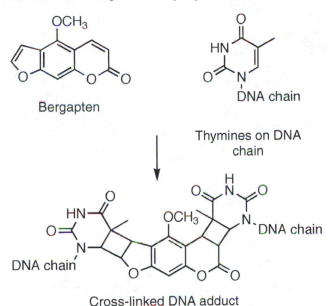

Bergapten

Thymines on DNA chain

Cross-linked DNA adduct

FIGURE 4.23. Bergapten reacting with DNA to form a cross-link.

sugar molecules, and *cyanogenic* means "cyanide generating." When an animal (or human) eats plant material containing a cyanogenic glycoside, enzymes in the plant (released as it is crushed) or digestive acid cause the cyanide ion to be released. The reaction is illustrated in Figure 4.24, part a, for sambunigrin, found in elderberry plants *(Sambucus nigra)*.

Cyanide is very toxic to all animals as it short-circuits the electron transport chain, which in effect prevents the organism from using oxygen. Symptoms of oxygen deprivation occur and, if the dose is sufficient, death follows. Prunasin is an epimer[14] of sambunigrin found in cherry-laurel water (from *Prunus laurocerasus*) which is occasionally used in pharmacy as a respiratory stimulant. In the 1970s a compound called amygdalin, which is a different glycoside of prunasin's aglycone, was formulated into a cancer drug named Laetrile, which caused a great deal of controversy. It was eventually shown to be completely ineffective (Figure 4.24, part b).

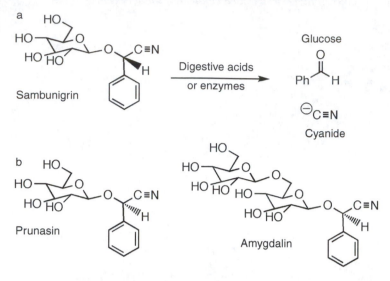

FIGURE 4.24. Cyanogenic glycosides. a: reaction of sambunigrin to release cyanide ion; b: other cyanogenic glycosides.

Glucosinolates

Glucosinolates are glycosides[15] of amino acid derivatives which also contain a sulfate group (SO_4). They are found primarily in the Brassicaceae, which is the plant family containing mustard, cabbages, and horseradish. When the seeds of black mustard *Brassica nigra)* are crushed, an enzyme called myrosinase is released and reacts with sinigrin, a glucosinolate present in the seeds. Myrosinase causes the sinigrin to be hydrolyzed[16] and rearranged to give a compound called allyl isothiocyanate, which is very reactive toward moist human mucous membranes (see Figure 4.25, part a). The allyl isothiocyanate is responsible for the gustatory properties of mustard and horseradish preparations, such as wasabi, a Japanese condiment served with sushi. Glucosinolates and the isothiocyanates derived from them are irritating but generally not toxic. In fact, ample data show that diets rich in vegetables containing glucosinolates have a significant cancer-protective effect. One example is sulforaphane, an isothiocyanate derived from a glucosinolate in broccoli and broccoli sprouts (Figure 4.25, part b). This compound activates certain en-

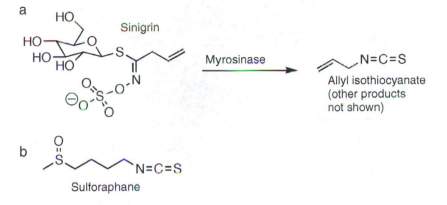

FIGURE 4.25. Glucosinolates. a: reaction to form an isothiocyanate; b: another isothiocyanate.

zymes that are able to detoxify toxic molecules, and it also induces cell death. These two modes of action make it a powerful cancer-protective agent.

Glycosides

Almost all plant molecules with a hydroxyl (alcohol) group are actually present in the plant as glycosides. Glycosides are formed when small hydroxyl-containing molecules are combined with one or more sugar (carbohydrate) molecules. The nonsugar portion is called the aglycone. Most often, an oxygen atom on the aglycone is the point of connection to the sugar, although occasionally one sees a nitrogen, sulfur, or carbon atom serve as the connecting atom.[17] Generally, glycosides are formed from specific sugars, including di- and trisaccharides, but glucose is the most abundant. Whatever the sugar molecule, the point of connection on the sugar is the carbon atom between the two oxygen atoms in the ring (shown by an arrow in Figure 4.26). If the molecule contains a sugar but is not connected to the rest of the molecule through the carbon between two oxygens, it is not a glycoside.

Many molecules have more than one atom to which a sugar can be attached, but not all such isomers may be found in nature, because the formation of glycosides is not random. Treatment with dilute acid

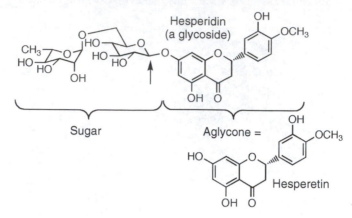

FIGURE 4.26. The relationship between glycosides and aglycones. The carbon noted with an arrow, and located between two oxygens on the sugar group, helps us recognize this as a glycoside.

breaks the bond between the sugar and the aglycone, a point that should be kept in mind when designing or evaluating isolation procedures (see Chapter 5). It is likely that many compounds isolated from plants were probably originally present as glycosides, but the sugar group was removed during the isolation process.[18] In many cases this is not just a technicality, because the biological activity is often due to the intact glycoside, not the aglycone.

Please bear in mind that the common names and terms used for these molecules are, unfortunately, very similar and confusing. For example, a glucoside is a glycoside in which glucose is the sugar. *Genin* is an older term for *glycoside,* and while it is no longer commonly used, the suffixes *nin* or *din* are often, but not always, found at the end of the name of a glycoside. The name of the corresponding aglycone is often only slightly different. The ending *oside* also designates a glycoside. An example should suffice to illustrate the challenges in deciphering these names. Two compounds are illustrated in Figure 4.26: hesperetin and hesperidin, which are flavonoids found in *Citrus* species. They are used for the treatment of poor venous circulation in the legs which leads to swelling (technically, chronic functional venous insufficiency). Hesperetin is the aglycone of hesperidin. The sugar is rutinose, so you could refer to hesperidin generically as a rutinoside, meaning a glycoside formed from rutinose.[19] Other examples of glycosides can be found in this chapter and are noted where they occur. (Careful study by those of you hoping for consistency will reveal just how inconsistent the name endings are.)

Isoflavones

Isoflavones are structural isomers of the flavonoids (see the previous section Anthocyanidins and Flavonoids in this chapter). Soybean products (e.g., tofu) are rich in isoflavones that mimic human estrogens and have been recommended as an alternative to synthetic hormones for the treatment of menopausal symptoms. The glycoside genistin is a good example (see Figure 4.27). Note that compared to the anthocyanidins and flavonoids (and the building blocks of the condensed tannins), the phenyl ring is located on an adjacent carbon.

Lignans

Lignans[20] are molecules assembled from building blocks composed of a benzene ring with a three-carbon chain attached to it. These building blocks are connected, at a minimum, by a bond between the second carbons of the three-carbon chains. Although many lignans have been discovered, few have found clinical use. A medicinally interesting example is the molecule podophyllotoxin (see Figure 4.28), isolated from the root of may apple (also called American mandrake or *Podophyllum peltatum*). This plant has been used historically by Native Americans for purging and in some cases as a poison. Its current use is for the external treatment of venereal warts caused by the papilloma virus; podophyllotoxin interrupts cell division very effectively and in fact is highly active against most viruses. Such an action

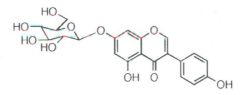

FIGURE 4.27. Genistin.

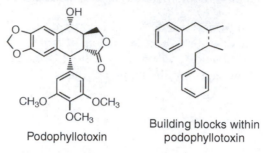

Podophyllotoxin

Building blocks within
podophyllotoxin

FIGURE 4.28. Lignans.

suggests a possible use as an anticancer agent. Podophyllotoxin proved to have too many side effects, but slight modifications of its structure in the lab have led to several potent compounds that are useful for specific types of cancers.[21]

Phenolic Compounds

Phenolic compounds is a frequently encountered term that applies to any molecule containing an aromatic ring with an alcohol on it (the simplest example, C_6H_5OH, is called phenol). Flavonoids, anthocyanidins, tannins, and lignans mentioned elsewhere in this chapter fall into this category. Phenolic *acids* include such molecules as gallic acid (see Figure 4.29, part a) which have both carboxylic acids and alcohols on an aromatic ring. The term *phenolic compounds* comes up frequently in Chapter 5's discussion of the antioxidant properties of plants.

Polyalkynes, Polyalkenes, and Related Compounds

Compounds containing multiple triple bonds (polyalkynes), multiple double bonds (polyalkenes), or combinations of these bonds are fairly unusual in nature and are found only in a few plant families. The two families of most importance are the Asteraceae (the sunflower family) and the Apiaceae (the parsley or carrot family). In addition to being structurally rather unique, many members of this group, or molecules derived from them, show interesting medicinal activity.

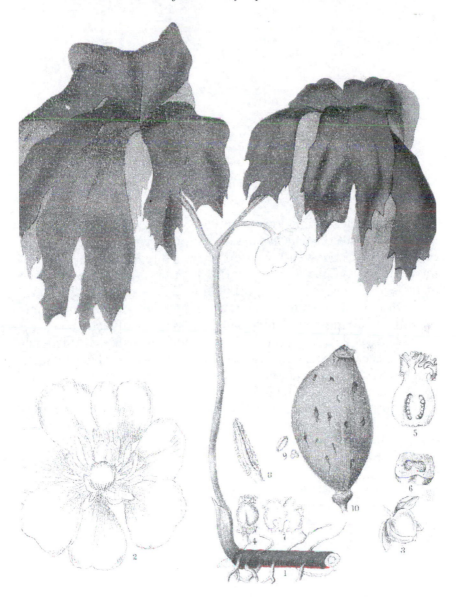

Podophyllum peltatum. (*Source:* Millspaugh, Charles F. *American Medicinal Plants: An Illustrated and Descriptive Guide to the American Plants Used As Homeopathic Remedies; Their History, Preparation, Chemistry and Physiological Effects.* New York: Boerick & Tafel, 1887. Vol. 1, pl. no. 17.)

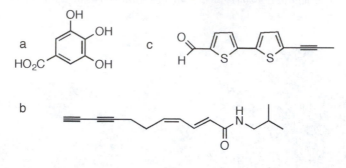

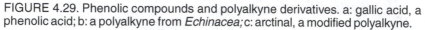

FIGURE 4.29. Phenolic compounds and polyalkyne derivatives. a: gallic acid, a phenolic acid; b: a polyalkyne from *Echinacea;* c: arctinal, a modified polyalkyne.

An economically important example is the genus *Echinacea* (the purple coneflowers), which is in the sunflower family.[22] Preparations of these species are well-known for their ability to stimulate the immune system to fight off cold and flu infections. At least two classes of molecules appear to be responsible for this activity: polysaccharides, discussed previously in the Carbohydrates section, and compounds containing both double and triple bonds (officially these are referred to as *enynes,* because of the alkene and alkyne functional groups). The compound shown in Figure 4.29, part b, which contains alkenes, alkynes, and an amide functional group, is typical of the types of compounds found in *Echinacea* species.

In some cases, plants modify the multiple bonds further to incorporate sulfur atoms. Arctinal, a compound found in burdock roots *(Arctium lappa)* appears to be one of several responsible for the antimicrobial and antifungal properties of that plant (see Figure 4.29, part c). Thiarubrine A, shown earlier in Figure 3.20, is another example in which sulfur has been incorporated into an unsaturated hydrocarbon chain. Many of these compounds are phototoxic (similar to the coumarins), but this activity is probably unrelated to the human medicinal uses previously mentioned.

Quinones

Quinones are compounds in which two ketone functional groups are embedded in an aromatic ring system. The simplest example, merely called quinone, illustrates this definition, but the medicinally interesting quinones are structurally more complex. Their chemistry is complex too—they are readily oxidized upon exposure to air and warmth and in some cases readily form dimers.[23] Thus, the storage and processing history of an herb containing quinones can significantly affect its medicinal properties. Glucofrangulin A (see Figure 4.30), a diglucoside, is found in the *dried* bark of buckthorn *(Rhamnus frangula)* and is one of several related compounds responsible for the laxative properties of this plant. Hypericin is found in St. John's wort *(Hypericum perforatum),* which was the second best selling herb in the United States in 1998; its structure was illustrated in Figure 1.1.

Tannins

Historically, tannins obtained from sources such as oak trees were used to "tan" or preserve animal skins and create leather, but modern methods of tanning make use of mineral substances for the most part. Tannins stabilize the collagen (a protein) in animal skins by working their way in between the collagen strands and then binding to the collagen and other proteins present in the skin. Tannins also precipitate most types of proteins. If taken orally or applied to the skin they produce astringency—a feeling of tightening and drying—due to the precipitation process. If significant quantities are taken orally, tannins can be quite hard on the stomach. Chemically, tannins fall into two classes, which are structurally quite different: the hydrolyzable tannins and the condensed tannins.

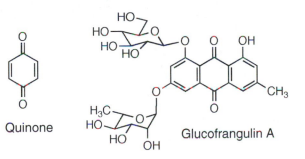

FIGURE 4.30. Quinones.

Hydrolyzable Tannins

Hydrolyzable tannins can be broken apart by the action of water.[24] They are esters of glucose combined with phenolic acids (phenols that also have carboxylic acids). Oenothein B (see Figure 4.31) is a molecule found in many plant species that has activity against the herpes simplex virus and the reverse transcriptase enzyme of HIV, as well as antitumor activity.

Condensed Tannins

Condensed tannins are also known as proanthocyanidins. The prefix *pro-* indicates that they can produce anthocyanidins, which are actually a type of flavonoid (see the section Anthocyanidins and Flavonoids).[25] They are polymeric, which means they are composed of chains of various lengths of a repeating unit; in this case the repeating unit is a flavonoid structure. The building blocks can be connected or linked to one another by different atoms. The polymeric nature and variety of linking schemes make it hard to study the condensed tannins, and thus only the simpler ones have been purified and studied. Cranberry juice (*Vaccinium macrocarpon*) is frequently sug-

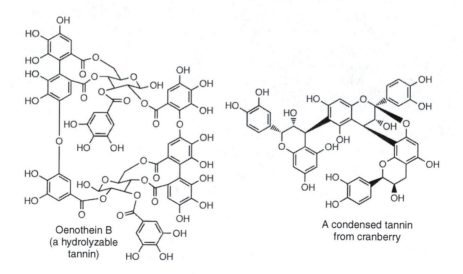

Oenothein B
(a hydrolyzable
tannin)

A condensed tannin
from cranberry

FIGURE 4.31. Tannins.

gested as an adjunct to antibiotic therapy for urinary tract infections. The compound shown in Figure 4.31 was recently isolated from cranberry juice and shown to inhibit attachment of bacteria to the cells lining the urinary tract. Note that it is composed of three identical flavonoid building blocks (linked in different manners) and hence could be called a trimer.

Terpenes

The terpenes are the largest group of plant secondary metabolites (the alkaloids are the second largest), and they exhibit a wide range of medicinal activities. In the material that follows I have chosen examples of compounds with demonstrated medicinal properties; keep in mind that many other terpenes have biological activity of other types. Terpenes are built from a specific five-carbon unit and, as a result, they generally have 10, 15, 20, 30, or 40 carbons in their structures. The isoprene rule was developed to help recognize terpenes via these five carbon building blocks (see Figure 4.32). This rule states that terpenes appear to be formed from head-to-tail combinations of isoprene units. Isoprene is *not* found in plants but serves as a simple aid to remembering the structural pattern. Some examples are shown in Figure 4.32 with the isoprene building blocks in bold. Terpenes are generally categorized according to the number of carbons in their skeletons, and the following discussion employs this convention.

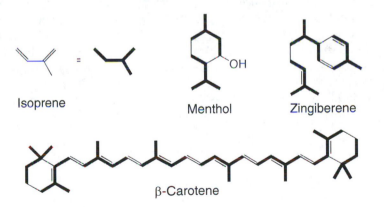

FIGURE 4.32. Isoprene and the application of the isoprene rule. Boldface indicates isoprene fragments within various terpenes.

Monoterpenes

Monoterpenes have ten carbons in their skeleton. Many are quite volatile and possess aromas ranging from pleasing to noxious. The essential oils are predominantly monoterpene mixtures. Iridoids are a specific type of monoterpene based upon a particular ring structure.

Essential oils. As a group, monoterpenes are the main components of essential oils obtained from plants by methods such as expression, extraction, or steam distillation, and they find use as medicines, flavoring agents, and perfumes.[26] Figure 4.33 gives a few examples of monoterpenes of medicinal interest. Keep in mind that the plants cited as the source of a particular molecule are generally not the only plant in which a given compound can be found. Further, since essential oils are always mixtures of many compounds, including some that are not terpenes, assigning medicinal activity to a single compound is often inappropriate. In the following cases I discuss the most abundant compound in the essential oil; this is by no means evidence that the most abundant compound is the active one.

Lavender oil (from *Lavandula angustifolia*) is an ancient herbal remedy with antiseptic and sedative properties. One of the main components responsible for improving sleep is linalool, which is found in high concentration in the oil. Eucalyptus oil, used in cough drops, contains a high percentage of 1,8-cineole, which is believed to be responsible for the expectorant and cough-suppressing activities of the oil. Peppermint oil (from *Mentha xpiperita*) has many of the same properties and is also useful in settling an upset stomach. Its main component is menthol. Sage species (*Salvia* spp.) contain a high amount of α-thujone; these herbs have been used to treat excessive sweating and digestive discomfort. α-Thujone is neurotoxic in high doses; it is found in wormwood (*Artemisia absinthum)* which was used to prepare the emerald green liquor absinthe. A condition known as absinthism was sufficiently common among artists, poets, and

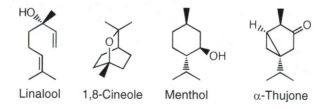

Linalool   1,8-Cineole   Menthol   α-Thujone

FIGURE 4.33. Monoterpenes typically found in essential oils.

those who traveled in similar circles that absinthe was banned in many countries early in the twentieth century.

Iridoids. The iridoids are a group of monoterpenes based upon the iridane ring system (Figure 4.34). Valtrate is one component of valerian root *(Valeriana officinalis)* that is recommended as a fairly strong sleep aid. Despite many investigations, no single component of valerian has been identified as the active ingredient. Note that valtrate is a triester; the ester groups should not be counted as part of the ten-carbon monoterpene skeleton.

Sesquiterpenes

Sesquiterpenes are composed of three isoprene building blocks, for a total of 15 carbon atoms. The most medicinally interesting types are the sesquiterpene lactones; *lactone* is a term referring to a cyclic ester group. Feverfew *(Tanacetum parthenium)* is an herb widely used for migraine relief. Its mode of action is not well understood, but parthenolide appears to play a role.[27] The Chinese herbal drug qing hao (sweet wormwood, *Artemisia annua*) is useful in treating malaria, and contains the compound qinghaosu which has an unusual oxygen-oxygen bond. Both compounds are shown in Figure 4.35.

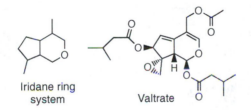

Iridane ring
system   Valtrate

FIGURE 4.34. Iridane monoterpenes.

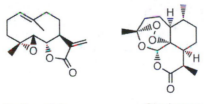

Parthenolide   Qinghaosu

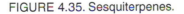

FIGURE 4.35. Sesquiterpenes.

Diterpenes

Unless you began reading right here, you should realize by now that diterpenes have a 20-carbon framework. The number of diterpenes with useful medicinal activity is limited, but the best example, paclitaxel, is a very important one (see Figure 4.36). Paclitaxel (Taxol) was originally isolated in extremely small quantities from the bark of the Pacific yew tree (Taxus brevifolia) found in old growth forests of the Pacific Northwest. When its great utility in treating advanced ovarian and breast cancers became clear, a race began to find other sources of the molecule, as obtaining it from its original source would literally wipe out the species.[28] Renewable sources were developed and paclitaxel became available in the early 1990s, though this molecule and its relatives are still receiving much research attention. As with some other examples we have seen, the C_{20} skeleton of paclitaxel is highly decorated, in this case with four ester groups whose carbons should not be counted in the total of twenty.

Triterpenes

Triterpenes possess a framework of approximately 30 carbons. Many are important as medicines or toxins. They fall into several categories which will be discussed separately.

Saponins. Saponins are glycosides of triterpenes that have soap-like properties. They are broadly distributed in the plant kingdom, and many of their aglycones have been used as starting materials for the synthesis of human hormones because of their structural similari-

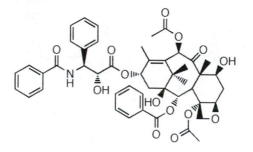

FIGURE 4.36. Paclitaxel, a diterpene.

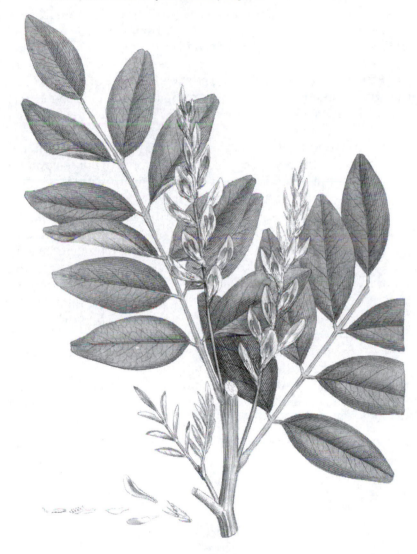

Glycyrrhiza glabra. (Source: Woodville, William. *Medical Botany* containing systematic and general descriptions, with pl.s of all the medicinal plants, indigenous and exotic, comprehended in the catalogues of the material medica; as published by the Royal College of Physicians of London and Edinburgh; accompanied with a circumstantial detail of their medicinal effects, and of the diseases in which they have been most successfully employed. London: printed and sold for the author by J. Phillips, 1793, Vol. 3, pl. no. 167.)

ties. A good example of this is diosgenin, which was isolated from the Mexican yam (*Dioscorea* spp.) and is a starting material for the synthesis of the hormones typically used in birth control pills.[29] Glycyrrhizin is a saponin from licorice root *(Glycyrrhiza glabra),* which is believed to be responsible for the anticough and antiulcer uses of the plant. Both compounds are shown in Figure 4.37. Ginseng *(Panax ginseng)* is another medicinally important plant that contains saponins.

Cardiac glycosides. Cardiac glycosides are named because of their potent effects on the heart; they increase the force of contraction and thus are useful in conditions such as congestive heart failure. They generally possess a narrow therapeutic margin, which means that the toxic dose is not that much larger than the therapeutic dose. Many of these compounds remain clinically important in spite of recent introductions of synthetic alternatives. Studies have shown that the aglycone actually provides the desired effects, but the entire glycoside is employed because of better solubility. The aglycones fall into two categories based primarily upon the size of the unsaturated lactone ring; examples are shown in Figure 4.38. The most significant plant both in terms of its clinical impact and its interesting history is the purple foxglove *(Digitalis purpurea),* which contains purpurea glycoside A. William Withering's investigations of the action of the foxglove are widely regarded as one of the first methodical studies of a plant drug. His *An Account of the Foxglove and Some of Its Medical Uses with Practical Remarks on Dropsy and Other Diseases* de-

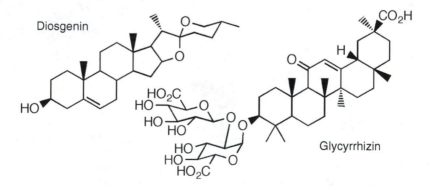

FIGURE 4.37. Saponins.

scribes how he treated patients suffering from dropsy, which is now generally called congestive heart failure. Withering experimented with different plant parts, preparations, and doses until he found a successful combination. Published in 1785, the book transformed the plant into a trustworthy mainstream medicine and provided a model for future medical studies of plants.

Tetraterpenes

The C_{40} tetraterpenes are of little medical value in the traditional sense. However, the carotenoids, compounds related to carotene, are of great interest as antioxidants (see Chapter 5). β-Carotene (see Figure 4.39) is a good example.

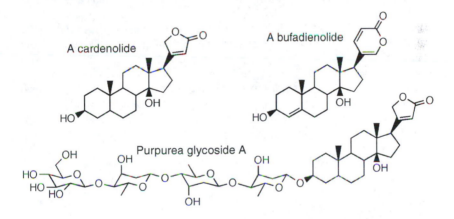

FIGURE 4.38. Cardiac glycosides.

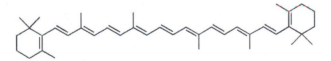

FIGURE 4.39. β-Carotene, a tetraterpene.

SUGGESTED READING

All texts on organic chemistry or introductory biochemistry have sections devoted to each of the four classes of primary metabolites described in this chapter. They should be consulted for more detailed information.

Ball, P. (2001). *Stories of the invisible: A guided tour of molecules.* New York: Oxford University Press. A very readable general discussion of the molecular world. Although it is not only about the molecules of life, a great deal of attention is given to them and the processes they mediate.

Bruneton, Jean (1999). *Pharmacognosy, phytochemistry, medicinal plants,* Second edition. Paris, France: Lavoisier. A technical yet reasonably accessible coverage of secondary metabolites. A good choice for additional information about any category of molecule discussed in this chapter.

Goodsell, D. S. (1998). *The machinery of life.* New York: Copernicus. An excellent, readable overview of how proteins, nucleic acids, and so forth assemble to create a functioning cell, capped off with a discussion of how viruses and poisons affect a cell.

Greenwood, David (1992). "The Quinine Connection." *Journal of Antimicrobial Chemotherapy* 30: 417-427. An interesting history of quinine, especially its role in World War II.

Hesse, Manfred (2002). *Alkaloids: Nature's curse or blessing?* Weinheim, Germany: Wiley-VCH. Although some of the information is quite technical, much of it is readable if you are seeking additional information about the alkaloids.

Widmaier, E. P. (2002). *The stuff of life: Profiles of the molecules that make us tick.* New York: Times Books.

Chapter 5

Chemical Behavior and Its Application to Medicinal Molecules

In this chapter, we apply what we have learned about structure and polarity in order to understand how medicinally active molecules can be isolated from plants. Then, we briefly consider the methods scientists use to identify and analyze medicinal molecules. Finally, we discuss the chemistry behind the functioning of antioxidants, an important class of chemicals which contributes significantly to human health.

ISOLATION OF MEDICINALLY ACTIVE SUBSTANCES

There is often great debate about whether one should use whole herbs for medicinal purposes or whether isolated and purified substances are preferable, especially for safety reasons. Such a question is really part of the larger debate between those who believe that all things natural are superior to all things synthetic. The nuances of the two points of view are worth investigating in detail elsewhere, but for now you should realize that even natural or organic forms of herbs have undergone some kind of extraction and processing. It is rare that one picks a few leaves and eats them directly. More likely, the leaves might be made into a tea. However, even such minimal processing as making a tea (or your morning coffee) constitutes a partial isolation and purification of a medicinal substance. No matter where you fall on the natural-versus-synthetic philosophical spectrum, you should know something about the processes by which medicinally active substances can be extracted from raw plant material. The polarity concepts that were discussed in Chapter 3 turn out to be the fundamental properties that control what happens in an extraction process.

Solubility and Extractions

Preparation of a medicinal tea would typically involve steeping the plant material in hot water. The potency of the tea would depend, in part, upon the temperature of the water, and how long the plant material soaked.[1] Other herbal preparations commonly seen include tinctures, which are extracts in alcohol, and ointments, where the active ingredient is dissolved or suspended in an oil or cream.

Consider what happens when you make a tea. A portion of leaves, possibly dried and crushed, is soaked for a few minutes in boiling water. Any molecules that will dissolve in the hot water do so, and they remain in the liquid to be consumed after the plant material is removed. The key question is, Which molecules will dissolve in hot water? After all, if the medicinally active molecules won't dissolve, the tea is not going to be effective. On the other hand, if they dissolve rather slowly, the medicinal effect (the strength of the tea) is going to depend greatly upon how hot the water was and how long the leaves were steeped.[2] Solubility is obviously an important concept to grasp. Chemists have a simple guideline to help us determine which molecules will dissolve. It is usually stated this way: "Like dissolves like," which means that polar solvents (liquids) will dissolve polar molecules. It could equally well be phrased as nonpolar solvents will dissolve nonpolar molecules. The concept is also embodied in the everyday saying, "Oil and water don't mix." Think of oil and vinegar salad dressing. The oil is composed of nonpolar molecules (see Chapter 4 under Lipids), while vinegar is mostly water. With its tetrahedral geometry and two very polar O–H bonds, water turns out to be one of the most polar molecules around, and oil is at the other extreme. Thus oil and water don't mix due to their differing polarities. When you shake the dressing vigorously to mix it, the two layers don't really mix but rather become suspended in each other as little droplets. This is called an emulsion.

In our tea-making example, we are using water as a solvent. Based on our "like dissolves like" guideline, we would expect that the water would extract and dissolve polar molecules in the leaves. If the medicinally active molecules are polar, then we would expect to get a medicinally active tea. If the medicinally active molecules are nonpolar, then our tea will be useless, and we should investigate other means of obtaining the active ingredient. I think you can see why our discussion of polarity was so important.

A familiar example of a medicinal tea would be the preparation of good old-fashioned tea from the leaves of *Camellia sinensis*. The caffeine (Figure 5.1, part a) contained in the leaves is very polar and readily dissolves in hot water. As a result, one gets a caffeine "buzz" from drinking tea. Different types of teas, such as black tea and green tea, result from different methods of aging the leaves. Though we are focusing on the extraction process, it is useful to keep in mind other similar variables that affect the quality of a medicinal plant product.

At the other extreme of solubility, consider capsaicin (Figure 5.1, part b), the component of chile peppers (*Capsicum* species) that is responsible for the burning sensation you feel when eating them. Capsaicin also has medicinal properties: it interferes with the pain sensation process (by several means). Ointments containing capsaicin have proven useful for the treatment of painful arthritic joints. Why is this administered as an ointment? In part, it is because the application is local in that the cream is rubbed into the skin of the joint, such as a knee.[3] However, a solubility issue is also at work here. Capsaicin is a nonpolar molecule, and ointments, creams, and oils are composed of nonpolar (oily) molecules which will dissolve the capsaicin. If you enjoy chile peppers for their culinary qualities, you might have heard that drinking milk can help quench the pain of a too-hot chile. If you try this, be sure to use whole milk, because it is the nonpolar fat in milk that can dissolve the capsaicin and carry it away from your burning mouth. Nonfat milk will be much less effective.

These examples illustrate how the polarity of the molecule and the polarity of the solvent must match if the molecule is to be extracted

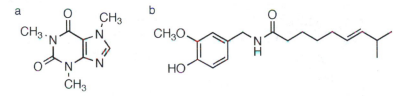

FIGURE 5.1. Examples of polar and nonpolar molecules. a: caffeine, a polar molecule; b: capsaicin, a nonpolar molecule.

into the solvent. In the scientific investigation of herbs, when one is looking for the active ingredient(s), it is usually desirable to use a range of solvents with differing polarities to extract the plant material. For example, let's say you identified a plant as being potentially useful medicinally.[4] After collecting some of the plant material, you might first soak (extract) it in hexane, $CH_3(CH_2)_4CH_3$, a very nonpolar solvent. This would dissolve any nonpolar molecules in the plant material. Next, you might filter off the hexane and save it, and then soak the remaining plant material in ethanol, CH_3CH_2OH. Ethanol is an alcohol of intermediate polarity, which would dissolve molecules of intermediate polarity. Finally, after filtering again, the plant tissue could be soaked in water, which would dissolve the very polar molecules. At this point, you would have four samples that you could test for medicinal activity; these are shown in Table 5.1.

The remaining plant tissue would generally be composed of "woody" material which, while potentially interesting, is practically speaking nearly impossible to study due to its insolublility. The other three samples each contain a variety of molecules within the indicated polarity range; literally thousands of molecules exist in any plant. It is an entirely different matter to determine if any of them are medicinally interesting. We will discuss how to do this later in this chapter. First, however, we need to be aware of another strategy for extracting molecules from a medicinal plant.

Using Acid-Base Behavior in Extractions

Two of the functional groups introduced in Chapter 2 behave in ways that make them very easy to extract from plants. The carboxylic

TABLE 5.1. Sequential extraction of a plant.

Extract	Contents
Hexane	Nonpolar molecules
Ethanol	Intermediate polarity molecules
Water	Polar molecules
Remaining plant tissue	Insoluble materials

acids (RCO_2H or $RCOOH$) function as mild or weak acids by giving up their proton:

$$RCO_2H \rightarrow RCO_2^- + H^+$$

The amines (R_3N) act as weak bases by accepting a proton:[5]

$$R_3N + H^+ \rightarrow R_3NH^+$$

Although important in other areas of chemistry, it is not the acid-base behavior *per se* that interests us right now but rather the effect of protonation/deprotonation on polarity, and therefore solubility. The carboxylic acid group, RCO_2H, is itself rather polar, but whether the whole molecule is polar will depend upon the nature of the R group, as discussed in Chapter 3. However, once the acid gives up its proton and the molecule becomes RCO_2^-, it is much more polar because of the full negative charge.[6] The same can be said of the amines—they are moderately polar (depending upon the structure of R), but when they accept a proton they become charged (R_3NH^+) and therefore much more polar. We can use this behavior to selectively extract these molecules.

This is best illustrated by the alkaloids. This large class of plant molecules is described in more detail in Chapter 4; for now we need to know that they are amines and often extremely potent as medicines or toxins. A specific example with an interesting history is the molecule coniine. Coniine is found in the poison hemlock plant, *Conium maculatum,* which, as the story goes, was used to poison the Greek philosopher Socrates. If you were studying poison hemlock (or any other alkaloid containing plant), you could selectively extract just the alkaloids by soaking the plant material in dilute acid. The dilute acid would protonate the coniine, making it much more polar and water soluble (see Figure 5.2).

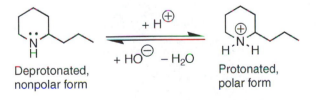

Deprotonated,   Protonated,
nonpolar form   polar form

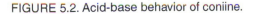

FIGURE 5.2. Acid-base behavior of coniine.

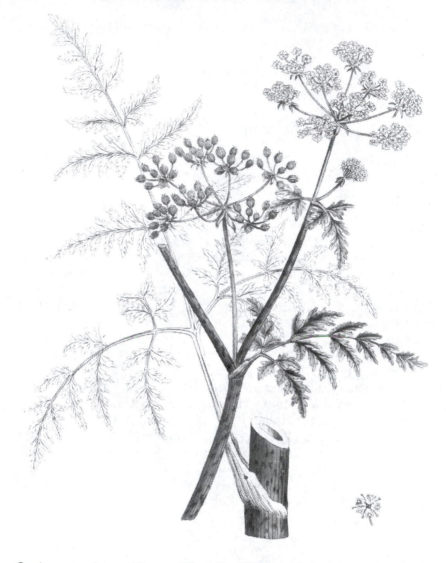

Conium maculatum. (*Source:* Woodville, William. *Medical Botany* containing systematic and general descriptions, with pl.s of all the medicinal plants, indigenous and exotic, comprehended in the catalogues of the material medica; as published by the Royal College of Physicians of London and Edinburgh; accompanied with a circumstantial detail of their medicinal effects, and of the diseases in which they have been most successfully employed. London: printed and sold for the author by J. Phillips, 1790, Vol. 1, pl. no. 22.)

To obtain pure coniine,[7] one would then filter off the plant residue to give an acidic solution containing protonated coniine. By adding a base such as sodium hydroxide to this solution, the acid would be neutralized, and the coniine deprotonated, reversing the previous reaction. At this point, the coniine is in its nonpolar, less-water-soluble form. Because it is no longer water soluble but is still in water, it might precipitate out of solution, in which case it can be filtered off to give pure coniine. More likely, one would take the basified solution and extract it with dichloromethane in a process known as liquid-liquid extraction. Dichloromethane, CH_2Cl_2, is a nonpolar molecule that will not mix with water. As it is nonpolar, it will dissolve the deprotonated, nonpolar form of coniine readily. Shaking the basic water solution of coniine with dichloromethane will move the coniine from the water, where it is not very soluble, into the dichloromethane, where it is very soluble. The dichloromethane can then be separated from the water and evaporated, leaving behind a sample of coniine. There is even a special piece of glassware designed for this extraction process called a separatory funnel. Its design makes it easy to shake the two liquids together and to separate the two liquids from each other. The entire extraction process is illustrated in Figure 5.3.

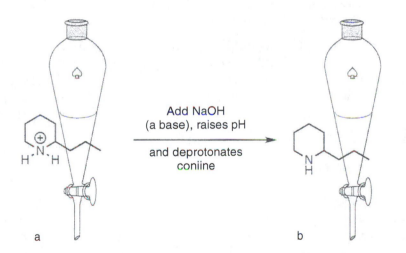

Add NaOH
(a base), raises pH

and deprotonates
coniine

a   b

FIGURE 5.3. Acid extraction of alkaloids. a: separatory funnel containing an acidic aqueous solution of coniine in protonated form; b: after adding a base, funnel now contains a basic aqueous solution of coniine in deprotonated form.

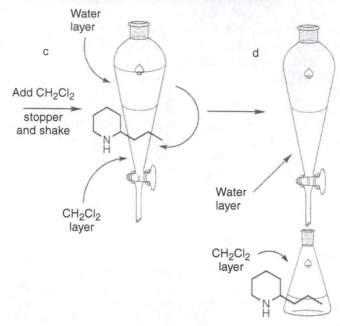

FIGURE 5.3 *(continued)*. c: after adding CH_2Cl_2, coniine moves from water to CH_2Cl_2 because it is more soluble in CH_2Cl_2 when deprotonated; d: the CH_2Cl_2 layer is drained into a flask, and can be evaporated to give coniine. The water layer is discarded.

Extraction by solvents of different polarity, or by using the acid-base behavior of molecules to vary their polarity, can accomplish a great deal of purification. However, because so many molecules are typically found in a plant, further treatment is usually necessary to obtain material that is pure. The most commonly used method, chromatography, is our next subject.

Chromatography

Chromatography comes from the Greek words meaning "to write or record with color," and, indeed, the early forms of chromatography were very colorful. In modern use, chromatography is a collection of closely related methods used to separate molecules. Chromatographic methods work because of the attractions molecules can exert on one another. Polarity is one reason for such an attraction—polar molecules are attracted to other polar molecules. This is the basis for the "like dissolves like" guideline noted earlier. Molecules can exert other types of attractions on one another, and we'll cover some of them in Chapter 6. However, polarity is a sufficiently broad concept that it will suffice to explain how chromatography works for our purposes.

A commonly used form of chromatography is thin-layer chromatography, more often referred to by its initials, TLC. In any chromatographic method, including TLC, there are two "parts" to the experiment: the stationary phase and the mobile phase. The stationary phase is some sort of material, generally a solid or gel, that is fixed in the experiment so that it does not move. In TLC, the stationary phase is a thin layer of silica (SiO_2) spread over a piece of stiff plastic or aluminum foil. This "plate," as it is called, is usually about the size of a microscope slide, although they can be made in any size.

The formula of silica, SiO_2, is a bit misleading. Rather than being composed of just three atoms, silica is composed of millions of silicon and oxygen atoms bonded together to form a three-dimensional framework; Figure 5.4 shows a two-dimensional view of silica (it's very difficult to draw a three-dimensional view of silica gel and still be able to see the part that is important in the TLC experiment).

In reality, on a molecular scale, the framework of silicon and oxygen atoms continues for a great distance in all directions, except at the surface (the arrows in the structure shown in Figure 5.4 should be taken to mean that the pattern of atoms repeats). The surface of the silica is the important part for explaining TLC. Note in Figure 5.4 that on the surface of silica are Si–OH groups, which we call silanols. Silanols are like the alcohol functional group in that they are very polar. This makes the *silicastationarphaseinTLCverpolar*   .

In a TLC experiment, one takes the plate coated with silica and "spots" it with a sample to be analyzed. Spotting is the process of placing a very small dot of a solution of chemicals to be analyzed on the plate, near one end. The solution of chemicals might be one of the

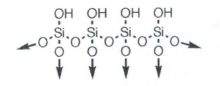

FIGURE 5.4. A two-dimensional view of silica gel.

extracts described in the previous section, such as the nonpolar extract of a medicinal plant. Or if you wanted to check the quality of a herbal capsule you had purchased, you could open the capsule, add some water or other solvent to the material, let it stand for a while to dissolve the compounds, and then spot the solution onto a TLC plate. Once the solution is spotted, the solvent evaporates, leaving a tiny sample of the compounds to be analyzed on the plate.

The next step in the experiment is to take the plate, spotted with the material to be analyzed, and stand it up in a jar that contains a small amount of solvent in the bottom, so that only the bottom edge of the plate is in the solvent. The solvent will wick up to the top of the plate in a few minutes; because the solvent is moving up the plate, it is called the mobile phase. In a standard TLC experiment, one can use a wide variety of solvents as the mobile phase. They may range from rather polar to rather nonpolar, but *compared to the silica gel stationary phase, the mobile phase is much less polar.*

The interesting part of TLC starts when the solvent, wicking up the plate, encounters the spot of chemicals to be analyzed. As the solvent front crosses the spot and continues to move upward, a competition of sorts begins. The molecules being analyzed have to make a decision, so to speak: either they "like" the mobile phase, or they "like" the stationary phase. I did not use the word *like* by accident here; essentially this is another "like dissolves like" situation. A less polar molecule will like the less polar mobile phase more, and move with it. A more polar molecule will like the very polar stationary phase more, and move more slowly. The net result is that nonpolar molecules will move farther up the plate than polar molecules. Assuming that the solution you are analyzing contains several compounds and that conditions have been chosen properly, each molecule will move to a different position.[8] When the solvent has made it up to the top of the plate, one removes the plate from the jar and the solvent is allowed to evaporate. Most compounds do not appear colored to the human eye, so some sort of visualization method has to be used to locate the compounds. The most common technique is to view the plate under ultraviolet light; most compounds will show up as dark spots.

TLC is great as a *qualitative* analysis method, used to get some idea of how many compounds are in a sample. If you are expecting something to be relatively pure, then you would expect to see one major spot on the plate, perhaps along with some minor spots. If you were analyzing a herb capsule, as mentioned earlier, and had a sample of authentic ingredient to use as a standard, then you could run your standard on the plate next to the material being tested. By comparing the spots from the authentic material with those from the capsule, you could estimate purity in a rough way. Such a situation is shown in Figure 5.5.

On the other hand, if you wanted to be *quantitative* to find out the exact amounts of each compound in your sample, TLC would not work well, because it is hard to measure the spots in a quantitative manner. However, one variation of TLC would allow you to be quantitative and would also allow you to work with much more material. In the technique called column or liquid chromatography, the stationary phase is still silica, but instead of a thin layer a lot of silica is packed into a tube through which the mobile phase flows. The sample is carefully layered onto the top of the bed of silica (the column), and solvent (mobile phase) is allowed to drip through the column. Components of the sample move through the column based on the same principles as in TLC; more nonpolar compounds move faster. The difference is that the TLC experiment is stopped when the solvent reaches the top of the plate. After allowing the solvent to evaporate, you view the plate, and observe a *spatial* separation of the com-

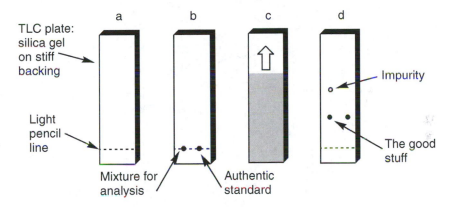

FIGURE 5.5. The TLC process. a: a light pencil line is drawn as a guide for placing the samples on the plate; b: dilute solutions of the mixture to be analyzed and a standard are spotted on the line using a very tiny tube; c: the plate is placed in a jar containing solvent (the mobile phase) so that the solvent wicks up the plate and past the spots; d: the plate is removed from the jar and the solvent allowed to evaporate. The spots are visualized with ultraviolet light or other means.

pounds. In column chromatography, mobile phase keeps flowing, and the molecules being analyzed eventually reach the end of the column and drip out with the solvent. This mobile phase, and any compounds it contains, is collected in a series of test tubes as it drips out. These are called fractions. Thus, column chromatography is really a *temporal* separation, because the different components reach the end of the column at different *times* (see Figure 5.6).

Once you have a series of fractions, you then have to figure out what, if anything, is in each of them. If you are incredibly lucky, the compounds might be colored and you can merely inspect the set of test tubes to find out which ones have something in them. A more general way to decipher the contents of the tubes is to perform TLC on each fraction. A large TLC plate is made in which each fraction is spotted in order along the pencil line. After developing the plate with mobile phase, evaporating the solvent, and visualizing, you might see something similar to the plate shown in Figure 5.7. In this example, three compounds were in the mixture analyzed. One of the compounds was obtained quite pure in fractions 4 through 7. These fractions can be pooled together and the solvent evaporated to give the sample. The other two compounds were not obtained completely

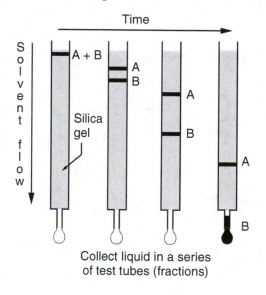

FIGURE 5.6. Column chromatography.

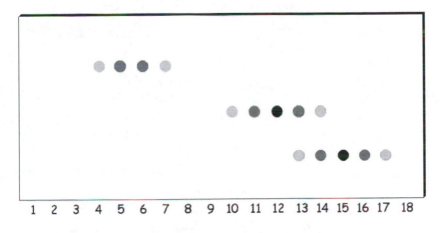

FIGURE 5.7. Analysis of chromatography fractions using TLC.

pure, as fractions 13 and 14 contain both compounds. However, one could pool fractions 10 through 12 to get pure material, and separately, pool fractions 15 through 17 to get the last compound pure. Fractions 13 and 14 could be subjected to further purification if desired.

To make this procedure as convenient as possible and truly quantitative, one can automate the column chromatography process and use some sort of detector instead of TLC to identify when compounds are exiting the column and going into the test tubes. The machine that does this is called a high performance liquid chromatograph (HPLC). A variety of detectors can be used with HPLC, and under the right conditions the detection process can be made quantitative. A typical HPLC system is shown in Figure 5.8. The process is virtually the same as manual column chromatography except for plumbing and the presence of a detector, which eliminates the need for a separate TLC analysis of the fractions. Instead, the detector measures some property of the molecules exiting the column, and converts this to an electrical signal. The result is a chromatogram which shows peaks when compounds leave the column. This can be used as a guide to the what is in the fractions. A typical chromatogram is shown in Figure 5.9.

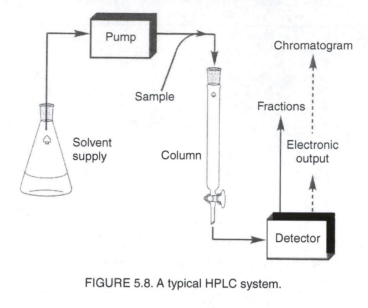

FIGURE 5.8. A typical HPLC system.

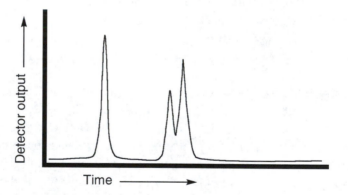

FIGURE 5.9. A typical HPLC chromatogram. This example corresponds to the TLC plate in Figure 5.7. One compound elutes quickly and is well separated; the two slower ones overlap.

Bioassays

HPLC and TLC are great methods to use to check the purity of chemical samples, especially when you have some idea in advance of what might be in the sample. However, if you are investigating a plant for interesting medicinal activity for the first time, those methods are of much less use because these techniques don't measure biological activity. For this purpose, you need to use a bioassay, which is a general term for methods of measuring biological response.

Let's say you have heard legends about the medicinal properties of some plant. You collect that plant and use solvents of different polarities to extract materials from the plant material (as described earlier in this chapter). You could use TLC to get an idea of how many compounds are in each extract and try to purify each of them, but that would be extremely time-consuming. In addition, the vast majority of molecules you would isolate would be of no medical interest. A much better strategy would be to subject each extract to a bioassay and determine if it has medicinal activity. This brings us to the chief advantage of using bioassays. If a particular extract has no biological activity, you don't need to continue to purify it. Throw it away and focus your efforts on extracts that do have biological activity. Any preliminary extract that does show activity would likely be subjected to column chromatography next, giving perhaps a couple dozen fractions. Each of these would then be bioassayed, and again, only those showing activity would be further purified. Whatever purification steps prove necessary, we only bother with the biologically active fractions. Eventually, we would hope to end up with one or more pure compounds with biological activity.

Using bioassays to guide your work greatly speeds up the process of finding new molecules of medicinal interest.[9] However, it is very important to realize that *the choice of bioassay determines what you will discover.* If you are bioassaying for blood-pressure-lowering activity, you will not discover molecules with anticancer properties. Because so many molecules are found in any plant, and so many possible biological activities can be measured, scientists won't be running out of plants to investigate for a long time. Even comparably well-studied plants may yield new medicines if investigated with a different bioassay.

So far I have referred to bioassays in a general way. When we get down to specifics, a tremendous variety of bioassays are possible that vary in the time it takes to conduct them, their expense, and the type of information you can get from them. On the simple, fast, and inexpensive end of the spectrum, there is McLaughlin's brine shrimp lethality assay. In this assay, brine shrimp larvae (a crustacean better known to many as "Sea-Monkeys") are subjected to solutions of plant extracts of various concentrations. After 24 hours of swimming in the plant extracts, the percentage of dead shrimp is determined. A higher percentage means greater biological activity. This assay has the significant advantages of requiring only readily available and inexpensive chemicals, and it takes only 24 hours to conduct. An important question to ask, however, is, What does it measure? Obviously, from the shrimps' point of view, it measures the ability of the extracts to kill shrimp larvae. In human terms, we don't really know what this means. We could reasonably speculate that brine shrimp larvae are rapidly growing and developing creatures, so any extract that kills them probably interferes with some aspect of cell growth and differentiation. In fact, it has been shown that many anticancer agents give a positive result in this assay, which is consistent with the model of cancer as a cell growing out of control. Nevertheless, because of the differences in organisms, it would be inappropriate to use the brine shrimp lethality assay as anything other than a preliminary screen for interesting biological activity.

Another simple bioassay is the zone of inhibition assay for antibiotic activity, which measures the bacterial killing power of a plant extract. A small circle of filter paper is soaked in plant extract and placed on a petri dish containing agar that has been uniformly inoculated with bacteria. The bacteria are allowed to grow for about 24 hours. During this time the extract diffuses into the agar around the disk. If the extract kills the bacteria, a clear zone around the disk will be seen where the bacteria were not able to grow. The larger this zone, the more powerful the killing ability of the extract. Such an experiment is shown in Figure 5.10.

At the other end of the spectrum are the assays available to pharmaceutical companies. These are typically very specific and very expensive. For instance, sophisticated assays that measure the activity of compounds against HIV in a test tube have been developed. Animals have been bred or genetically engineered to have asthma, diabetes, high blood pressure, and any number of human diseases. Not only are the animals expensive to develop and house but the assays are generally time-consuming. Most pharmaceutical companies make thousands of new compounds yearly, but it is impractical to test all of them using all of the in-house assays. Somewhere in between these

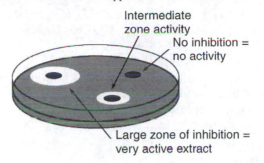

FIGURE 5.10. Zone of inhibition assay for antibiotic activity.

two extremes are cell culture assays, in which cells from particular organs are grown and dosed with plant extracts.

Finally, I should mention that any bioassay must be conducted on large numbers of creatures in order to have statistical significance. If the assay involves bacteria that can readily be grown by the billions, there's no problem. However, if the test animal is a genetically engineered rabbit, the cost can be extremely high. So many test animals are needed because although most animals of a given kind look the same, they are not really the same genetically, which means they are not the same biochemically. Humans are a good example: some people are allergic to certain drugs; others aren't. Some people are lactose intolerant and others aren't, and so on. These types of biochemical variations have a genetic basis, and one needs large numbers of individuals so that the full range of genetic variability is included in the trial. In the United States a long series of clinical trials (essentially bioassays on humans) are required before a drug is approved. (Human clinical trials occur only after many tests in animals.) Even so, in recent years several drugs have been pulled from the market because of problems discovered *after* a successful clinical trial. Fen-Phen is widely known example. The "fen" in the mixture is fenfluramine, which was found to cause damage to heart valves. This very serious side effect was apparently missed in the clinical trials because it is rare, and it wasn't until the drug became extremely popular and millions of people were using it that the problem became apparent. Vioxx is another widely used drug for which problems were discovered after approval.

ANALYSIS AND IDENTIFICATION
OF MEDICINAL MOLECULES

After isolating, by whatever means, molecules with medicinal activity, it eventually becomes important to know the structure of the molecules you have found. Without the structure, we won't be able to make hypotheses about how the molecule works, and thus we won't be able to modify it and make it work better. Likewise, you will need ways to analyze the molecules in a quantitative manner. Spectroscopy is the means to both of these ends.

Spectroscopy

Spectroscopy is the study of how light interacts with molecules. The definition of light, however, is not restricted to light as perceived by human eyes. The light we humans see is merely one kind of electromagnetic radiation. Others include such apparently different kinds as cellular phone waves, cosmic rays, and microwave radiation (from ovens or radar installations). Certain types of electromagnetic radiation can be used to help determine the structure of molecules by means we shall explore momentarily.

Before going into any particular method, however, let's remind ourselves of the problem we are trying to solve. In Chapter 2 we discussed structural isomerism, the situation in which molecules have the same molecular formula but different connectivities. We saw that for even relatively few atoms, the range of structures possible was rather large: for instance, $C_5H_{10}O$ allows for many possible connectivities or structures. Spectroscopy is used to determine which of the many possible structures is in fact the actual structure. Many types of spectroscopy are available; we'll look at two closely and mention some others briefly.

Infrared Spectroscopy

In infrared (IR) spectroscopy, light (radiation) within a certain frequency[10] range hits a molecule and causes the bonds in the molecule to vibrate. A good mental picture of the effect is to think of the bonds as springs, which may be very stiff or very flexible depending upon the type. A stiff bond would correspond to a strong bond. The strength of the bond depends upon the atoms involved in the bond and whether the bond is single, double, or triple. Chemists must be a lucky bunch, because it turns out that a wide variety of bond types require very specific frequencies to cause them to vibrate. The result is that one can compare the "peaks" seen in an IR spectrum with a table of typical vibration frequencies and learn a lot about the structure of a molecule. Because each functional group contains certain types of bonds, we typically use IR spectroscopy to determine which functional groups are present in an unknown molecule. A correlation table of functional groups and frequencies is given in Table 5.2.

The process is so simple that we can go right to an example. The IR spectrum of an unknown molecule with formula $C_5H_{10}O$ is shown in

TABLE 5.2. IR correlation table.

Group	Peaks	Comments
Alkanes	C–H stretch *below* 3,000	Present in virtually all molecules
Alkenes	C–H stretch *above* 3,000	
	C=C stretch 1,600-1,675	
Alkynes	≡C–H stretch 3,300	Infrequent
	C≡C stretch 2,150	Sharp, moderate intensity (doesn't generally overlap with C≡N)
Aromatics	=C–H stretch *above* 3,000	
	C=C stretch 1,600 and 1,450	
Alcohols	O–H stretch 3,200-3,500	Very strong, broad
Amines	N–H stretch 3,200-3,500	1° amines 2 bands 30 apart; 2° weak
Nitriles	C≡N stretch 2,250	Very sharp, moderate intensity (doesn't generally overlap with C≡C)
Carbonyls (values ± 5-10) all carbonyls are *strong*	ester 1,735	
	aldehyde 1,725	Check also for C–H @ 2,750
	ketones 1,715	
	acids 1,710	Very broad; also has O–H
	amides 1,690	Might have N–H

Note: Frequencies are approximate and given in cm^{-1} (wavenumbers).

Figure 5.11. Let's tour the parts of the spectrum and then figure out which functional groups are present in the molecule. The horizontal axis of the spectrum is the frequency axis, measured in a unit called wavenumbers. When attempting to determine what functional groups are present, we look primarily at the peaks above about 1,500 wavenumbers (cm⁻¹).[11] The vertical axis of the spectrum describes the intensity of the peaks, and in IR spectroscopy, *peaks point down* (this results from how the first instruments were built). When looking at an IR peak, there are three things to note: frequency, intensity, and shape. Some peaks are very broad, while some are sharp. Such information can be quite useful and is noted in the table. In the example in Figure 5.11, you can see the following peaks above 1,500 cm⁻¹:

- A broad peak at 3,345 cm⁻¹
- A group of several peaks, the largest at 2,872 cm⁻¹

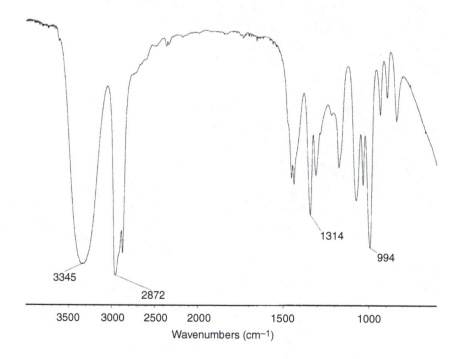

FIGURE 5.11. IR spectrum of an unknown sample.

Comparing the spectrum to the correlation table, we can see that the group of peaks around 2,900 cm^{-1} is due to the carbon-hydrogen bonds. Since most molecules have such bonds, this is not of much use, although we would not want to mistake the CH peak for something else. The peak at 3,345 cm^{-1}, however, is very useful, as it tell us we have an alcohol or amine group in our molecule.

If we turn now to analyzing our molecular formula, $C_5H_{10}O$, we see that there is no nitrogen in the formula, so an amine functional group is out of the question.[12] Continuing, we can exploit the information in the molecular formula further using a concept called the index of hydrogen deficiency or IHD. For every IHD unit in a molecule, there is one ring or one double bond in the structure. A triple bond counts as two IHD units. Thus, a formula with an IHD of three could mean the structure has three rings, or alternatively three double bonds, or a triple bond plus a ring, and so on. This concept is very useful in helping determine a structure, particularly if you have other information that you can use. Here is the method of calculating the IHD:

$$\text{IHD} = \#\,C - (0.5\times \quad \#\,H) + (0.5\times \quad \#\,N) + 1$$

If you apply this formula to the mysterious $C_5H_{10}O$, you'll see that the IHD for this formula is $5 - 5 + 1 = 1$, which means that the molecule has either one ring or one double bond. We could have discovered this by drawing possible structures manually. However, as molecules get larger the advantages of using the IHD multiply. It is much easier to calculate the IHD for a formula such as $C_{17}H_{23}NO_3$ (atropine from Figure 2.6) rather than first attempting to draw some isomers, because you will have some ideas about parts of the structure. By calculating the IHD, you save a lot of aggravation.[13]

We are left then with the conclusion that our molecule must contain an alcohol functional group. (Some other oxygen-containing functional groups are ethers, aldehydes, and ketones, which would be consistent with the molecular formula but not the IR spectrum.) The IHD, which works out to be one in this case, means there is either a ring or a double bond present in the molecule. What are the possible structures? Working from $C_5H_{10}O$, the knowledge that an alcohol is present, the rules of bonding, and the index of hydrogen deficiency, we can come up with some possible structures. A few are shown in Figure 5.12. Although the structures show variety, still other possible structures are not illustrated. Which one is correct? Is the correct structure even in the figure? Based upon a more careful examination of the IR data, we can narrow the field a little. If you consult the IR correlation chart, you'll see that the presence of an alkene (double bond) would produce two types of peaks *that are not in our spectrum:* a CH peak at slightly higher than 3,000 cm^{-1} and a peak due to the alkene C=C bond in the range of 1,600 to 1,675 cm^{-1}. With this approach, we are studying the possible structures and asking what IR spectrum would they produce. This strategy complements our first approach, which was to look at the IR spectrum and infer what functional groups were present. Using this sort of logic, we can eliminate any structure with an alkene, because there is no evidence in the IR spectrum for an alkene. Unfortunately, that still leaves many possible structures which possess a ring. If we were able to look up reference spectra of each molecule with a ring and compare it to our spectrum, we could probably figure out which structure we had. However, reference spectra are not always available. Instead, if we use our IR data with other spectroscopic methods, we might be able to determine the actual structure.

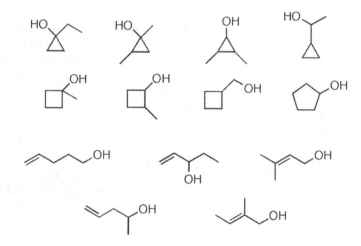

FIGURE 5.12. Some isomeric structures with formula $C_5H_{10}O$ (which has IHD = 1).

Carbon-13 Nuclear Magnetic Resonance

Carbon-13 (C-13) nuclear magnetic resonance (NMR) is a type of spectroscopy that gives us different information about structure than IR spectroscopy does. The theory behind NMR is complicated, so I will say only a little about it, by picking apart its name. The word *nuclear* tells us that the nucleus of the atom is involved. Carbon-13 is a particular type of carbon atom[14] that has six protons and seven neutrons in its nucleus. *Magnetic* tells us that the nucleus of carbon-13 acts like a tiny magnet, and *resonance* is a term which implies that two things are matched or tuned to work together in some way. Putting these terms together, we can give a simple summary of NMR theory by saying that the instrument is tuned to observe the magnetic behavior of the carbon-13 nucleus. You may actually be familiar with an NMR instrument, but under the name MRI—magnetic resonance imaging. This is a medical imaging technique that uses the same principle as NMR. The word *nuclear* was removed from the name because of the negative connotations of the term.[15]

Let's go straight to how we can use C-13 NMR data to help find the structure of a molecule. A C-13 NMR spectrum of the same sample we used for our IR example (from Figure 5.11) is shown in Figure 5.13. The horizontal axis is called the chemical shift and is measured in parts per million (ppm). The vertical axis corresponds to peak strength; peaks point up in NMR spectroscopy. You'll note that the peaks in C-13 NMR are very narrow and that there is sometimes "noise" in the baseline.

When interpreting this data, look for two things: how many peaks there are and their chemical shift values (we don't measure peak strength or height in C-13 NMR). The number of peaks in the spectrum tells us the number of unique carbon atoms in the structure. This is not always the same as telling us the number of carbons present. If there is any symmetry in the structure, the number of peaks in the C-13 spectrum will be less than the number of carbons present. Symmetry means that the molecule can be cut into two equal halves, three equal parts, etc. In some ways it may be easier to define asymmetry, which would be the lack of any kind of equality within different parts of a molecule.[16]

The chemical shift of each peak tells us a little about the type of carbons present, as shown in Table 5.3. In the C-13 spectrum of our

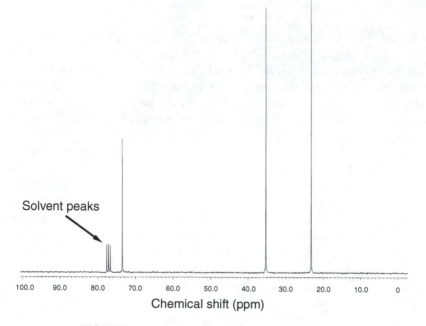

Solvent peaks

Chemical shift (ppm)

FIGURE 5.13. C-13 NMR of an unknown sample.

TABLE 5.3. C-13 NMR shifts.

Type of carbon	Shift (ppm)
Saturated carbons[a]	0-80
Double bonded, including benzene rings	105-160
Triple bonded	
$C\equiv C$	75-95
$C\equiv N$	115-130
Carbonyls	
Ketone	205-230
Aldehyde	185-205
Carboxylic acid	170-185
Ester and amide	160-175

[a]An N, O, or any electronegative element attached to a saturated carbon generally moves its shift to a higher number within this range.

unknown, you can see a total of three peaks (in addition to the solvent peaks, which are marked). This tells us that there are three unique carbon environments in our molecule. Because we know our molecule has five carbons, and the C-13 spectrum has three peaks, we know there must be some symmetry in our molecule, otherwise there would be five peaks in the spectrum. This will be a big help in narrowing the list of possible structures.

Turning to the chemical shift, we see that all the peaks in the spectrum are in the range expected for saturated (singly bonded) carbons. One peak, the one at about 73 ppm, would be consistent with a carbon that has the oxygen atom attached to it. To cross-check our conclusion from the IR spectrum that an alkene is not possible, note that there are no C-13 peaks in the range expected for an alkene carbon (105-160 ppm; this region was not plotted in Figure 5.13 as there were no peaks).

At this point, our analysis of the data allows us to make the following statements about our unknown compound:

- It has a molecular formula of $C_5H_{10}O$.
- An alcohol (–OH) is present.
- Only saturated carbons are present.
- Symmetry is present.
- Index of hydrogen deficiency is one, implying a ring or double bond (but the latter has been ruled out).

Of the ring structures in the chart earlier, the ones shown in Figure 5.14 have some element of symmetry in their structures (I have marked the approximate line of symmetry with a dotted line, but making a physical model may help you see how flexibility affects the apparent symmetry). Structures B and F have three unique carbon environments, and all of the others have four unique carbon environments.[17] Thus, either B or F must be the correct structure. To decide between these two, we would need still more data, but as you can see, we have narrowed a very long list of possible structures to just two.

Mass Spectrometry

Another tool frequently used to help determine structure is mass spectrometry (MS). This is a very powerful technique, but skill in

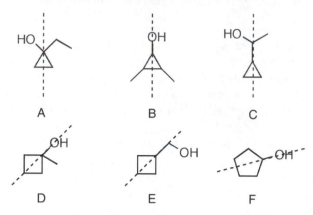

FIGURE 5.14. Some $C_5H_{10}O$ isomers with symmetry (indicated by dotted line).

interpreting the data takes quite some time to develop, so we won't go into detail. In some ways the experiment is pretty simple: your molecule is blasted with high energy electrons, and it falls to pieces. Studying the pieces that result can tell the experienced chemist something about the functional groups present, and whether or not bromine, chlorine, or nitrogen are present. And it can reveal the molecular mass of the molecule. The molecular mass can be very useful if you don't know the formula of the molecule. For example, if your molecule has a molecular mass of 80, it's impossible for there to be more than six carbon atoms in the molecule, because six carbons would have a mass of 72, while seven carbons would weigh more than 80. In fact, if there were exactly six carbons, a possible formula would be C_6H_8. However, C_5H_4O also has a mass of 80. I think you can see how mass spectroscopy can be used to put a limit on the possible structures, but it is rarely used by itself.

Mass spectrometry is a very sensitive technique—probably the most sensitive analysis method we have routinely available. It is used extensively in the environmental field and in forensic work, including monitoring athletes for drug use. So, besides being used to help with structure determination, the mass spectrometry experiment can also readily be made quantitative. Because of this, mass spectrometry is frequently used as a detection method in chromatography. We shall return to this in just a moment.

Chromatography As Means of Quality Control

Because we now know something about spectroscopy, I want to return to the topics of chromatography and analysis. An important issue in the marketing of herbs is standardization and quality control. Because herbs are generally sold as whole or partially processed material, and because growth conditions and plant genetics can affect the amount of active ingredient, we need to have some way to know how much active ingredient is in the product. This requires a method of analysis, and many methods of analysis rely on the spectroscopic techniques we've just covered.

Although TLC does not lend itself well to quantitative work, it is still used as a means of quality control.[18] Conditions have been worked out for many of the major herbal drugs so that one can determine whether the active ingredient is present and, in some cases, whether certain adulterants or undesirable compounds are present. Recall that in order to visualize the spots in a TLC experiment, one often views the plate under ultraviolet light. This is actually a form of spectroscopy; UV light is a particular set of wavelengths, and the compounds are absorbing some of the light that hits them, giving rise to various colors.

In HPLC, UV spectroscopy is frequently used as a detection method, and the process can be set up to be very quantitative. As the mobile phase flows out of the column, it passes through a chamber through which UV light also passes. If a compound is in the mobile phase at a particular time, it can absorb some of the UV light, and the amount absorbed can be electronically detected. If you have an authentic sample of the material, you can put known amounts of the compound through the system and measure the response. By doing this with several different amounts, one can develop a calibration curve which can be used to determine exactly how much of a compound is present in an unknown sample. An example of such a calibration curve is shown in Figure 5.15.

Another important type of chromatography frequently used to analyze herbal products is gas chromatography-mass spectrometry (GC-MS). Gas chromatography is very similar to HPLC, in that the sample flows with the mobile phase through a tube. However, in GC, the tube is extremely narrow and long, and its walls are coated with a gel that functions as the stationary phase. The mobile phase is helium gas

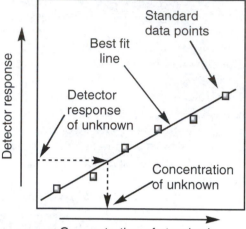

FIGURE 5.15. A typical calibration curve as used with HPLC or GC-MS. The standard data points are the responses from a set of prepared standards of known concentration.

flowing through the tube. The sample to be analyzed is injected into a heated zone, which causes it to turn to a gas. It then flows through the tube along with the helium gas. The more the compound interacts with the gel on the walls (the stationary phase), the slower it moves through the system. Upon reaching the end of the column, the sample moves directly into a mass spectrometer for detection. As for HPLC, known amounts of authentic compound can be used to develop a calibration curve. Table 5.4 summarizes what we have said about the different chromatographic methods.

ANTIOXIDANTS AND REACTIVE OXYGEN SPECIES: CHEMICAL REACTIONS AFFECTING HEALTH

Let thy food be thy medicine, and thy medicine be thy food.

Hippocrates (460-377 B.C.E.)

Antioxidants are molecules generally found in plants that can dramatically affect human health by intercepting another class of mole-

TABLE 5.4. Chromatographic methods.

Method	Scale: purpose	Stationary/ mobile phase	Nature of separation
TLC (thin-layer chromatography)	Small: qualitative inspection of mixtures	Silica gel/ solvent	Compounds move to different positions (spatial)
HPLC (high performance liquid chromatography)	Small → large: analyze or purify compounds	Silica gel/ solvent	Compounds exit column at different times (temporal)
Column chromatography	Medium → large: purify compounds	Silica gel/ solvent	Compounds exit column at different times (temporal)
GC-MS (gas chromatography-mass spectrometry)	Small: analyze something quantitatively	Gel/ helium gas	Compounds exit column at different times (temporal)

cules called reactive oxygen species. Reactive oxygen species are a normal part of human biochemistry, but a great quantity of data support the idea that an *excess* of reactive oxygen species plays an important role in many diseases. For instance, part of our immune system uses reactive oxygen species to destroy invading bacteria and viruses. However, if the immune response gets out of balance, the reactive oxygen species involved can do a great deal of "collateral" damage and cause inflammation—for instance, the redness and swelling seen around an infected cut. Scientists believe that many people live in a state of chronic inflammation caused by reactive oxygen species. The chronic inflammation they produce is believed to be the underlying cause of many cancers, as well as a whole spectrum of events we associate with aging, such as poor memory and muddled thinking, cataract formation, cardiovascular problems, and immune system decline. Although many diseases are believed to have links to an excess of reactive oxygen species, we shall focus on a well-documented case, atherosclerosis or hardening of the arteries, after we examine the basic chemical issues.

To understand how reactive oxygen species can cause damage, and therefore how antioxidants can intercept reactive oxygen species, we need to know something about each of them and their chemical reactions. We'll begin by defining what we mean by reactive oxygen species and then looking at a few principles governing chemical reactions in general.

What Are Reactive Oxygen Species?

Reactive oxygen species (ROS) is a term that, taken literally, includes molecules containing oxygen in a reactive form.[19] We will discuss the concept of reactivity momentarily; for now, let's name and describe the most important *primary* ROS (see Table 5.5). By using the term *primary,* I am indicating that these are the ROS originally formed by biological processes. Later we will see that these primary ROS can give rise to other types of ROS through subsequent reactions.

Two of the molecules in Table 5.5 have unusual arrangements of their electrons, which contributes to their reactivity. Superoxide and hydroxyl radical belong to a group of molecules known as free radicals, which are defined as molecules with an unpaired electron. To have an unpaired electron, a molecule must have an odd number of electrons. In addition to the unpaired electron, free radicals can possess a formal charge as well. The complete Lewis structures of hydroxyl radical and superoxide are also given in the Table 5.5, as are condensed formulas which are more typically seen. In the condensed formulas we draw the unpaired electron as a dot, as we do any electron; this emphasizes and reminds us of its reactive nature.

TABLE 5.5. Primary reactive oxygen species.

Name	Lewis structure	Condensed formula
Superoxide	$\cdot \ddot{O} - \overset{..}{O} \overset{\ominus}{:}$	$O_2^{\cdot -}$
Hydrogen peroxide	$H - \ddot{O} - \ddot{O} - H$	H_2O_2 (HOOH)
Hydroxyl radical	$H - \ddot{O} \cdot$	$HO^{\cdot}$

The term *free radical* indicates that these species are free to move around and react. There are also "caged" radicals, which are somehow trapped in the area in which they were created. A caged radical is generally not very reactive because it is immobilized within a limited area and thus cannot readily find a reaction partner. Free radicals can be quite reactive, but they can also be rather sluggish; reactivity is discussed more in the next section.

Finally, ROS are often characterized as oxidizers or oxidants (in contrast to *anti*oxidants). In chemistry, oxidation refers in part to reactions that add oxygen atoms to a molecule. However, there are several ROS for which oxidant is not a good description of their behavior, so ROS is a better, more encompassing term.

Chemical Reactivity

To understand the behavior of ROS and antioxidants, we need to have some appreciation of what is meant by *reactivity* in the chemical sense. In the usual usage of the word, a reactive molecule is one that reacts *quickly*. It is unwise, however, to merely describe a certain molecule as reactive, because the chemical or biochemical environment in which it exists will greatly influence its reactivity. Furthermore, the reactions we are interested in always involve another molecule, so when we speak of reactivity, we need to emphasize *with what*. Regardless of the reaction partner, however, reactivity will also depend upon a number of other factors. For instance, almost all reactions go faster at higher temperatures, because the molecules are moving faster and thus carry more energy. Reactivity generally depends greatly upon the concentrations of the reactants; usually a higher concentration of reactants means a faster reaction.[20] Finally, the solvent in which the reaction is run, other molecules that might be present, and so forth, can affect reactivity. If all these variables can be controlled, as they might be in a test tube experiment (the so-called in vitro or "in glass" experiment), then we can make meaningful comparisons about reactivity, at least under the specified conditions. What we are really interested in, though, is what occurs in a cell (in vivo, or "in life"). Because a cell contains so many different molecules, it is difficult to control all the variables that might affect reactivity. This makes comparisons of reactivity more difficult in the situations that are of greatest interest, but such is often the case in science.

I've defined reactivity as how quickly or how fast a molecule reacts. The chemist calls this the *rate of reaction*. The rate concept refers to the idea that a certain number of events are happening in a fixed period of time. If your car is traveling at 32 miles per hour (mph), this is a rate: 32 miles are traveled in one hour. Chemically, we might say that a certain number of molecules react per second. Besides the rate of reaction, you will sometimes hear the term *halflife* used to describe how fast a molecule reacts. The half-life of a chemical is the amount of time required to use up half the chemical present during a reaction. A shorter half-life (i.e., a smaller number) means the reaction is occurring faster. The half-life of some important ROS are given in Table 5.6, which includes not only the primary ROS mentioned earlier but also some secondary ROS.

Another useful thing to keep in mind is that reactivity is one side of the coin whose other side is *selectivity*. A highly reactive molecule is not very selective in what it reacts with. On the other hand, an unreactive molecule is quite selective. Put another way, a highly reactive molecule will react with many different molecules because it has lots of energy. If the other molecules are low on energy, the highly reactive one can supply it and make a reaction possible. A less reactive, less energetic molecule has to wait for a partner that has some pretty weak bonds to attack, and hence is more selective. Reactivity and control are also related concepts from a chemist's perspective. A highly reactive molecule is hard to control. To visualize this concept, consider how you might paint an old Victorian house with lots of de-

TABLE 5.6. Half-lives of important ROS.

ROS species	Half-life
HO•	10^{-9} seconds
L•	10^{-8} seconds
LO•	10^{-6} seconds
O_2•−	10^{-5} seconds
LOO•	7 seconds
H_2O_2	Several minutes

Note: 10^{-9} seconds = 0.000000001 seconds or one-billionth of a second; L represents a fragment of a lipid molecule.

tailed woodwork. A spray gun powered by compressed air would not be a good choice for painting the trim pieces—the paint would go all over the place. Instead of a too-reactive, hard-to-control power sprayer, you would probably want to use a small paintbrush for those detailed areas. In the context of our discussion, a highly reactive ROS will be not be very selective in what it reacts with—it will damage a variety of molecules and the cell will not be able to control it very well. Hydroxyl radical, with its very short half-life, is an example of a very reactive, hard-to-control ROS. In contrast, the lipid peroxy radical LOO• (the • represents and emphasizes the unpaired, reactive electron) is much longer lived, less reactive, and easier to control.

Before closing this section, I should clarify a term I snuck into the previous paragraphs—energy. I implied that a reactive molecule is an energetic molecule, and this is certainly true. But scientists use the term *energy* in several different ways, so we should explore these briefly. The energy inherent *in a single molecule* is composed of two kinds: kinetic energy, which comes from the motion of the molecule, and potential energy, which depends upon the strength of the bonds holding the molecule together. The energy *of a reaction,* on the other hand, depends upon the *differences* in energy between the reactants and products. Kinetic energy depends only upon temperature, so if we are talking about biochemical reactions occurring at a fixed 37°C, then the total kinetic energy doesn't change during a reaction, only the potential energy. A reaction in which the changes in bonding (and the related potential energy) result in energy being *released* are considered favorable.

Now here's the catch and why you must listen carefully when someone uses these terms: *an energetically favorable reaction may or may not occur.* Whether or not it will occur depends upon its *rate,* that is, the reactivity we just discussed. Many reactions would give off a lot of energy (be favorable) if they happened, but they are so slow to react that, in effect, nothing happens. For instance, the reaction of hydrogen gas with oxygen gas is energetically extremely favorable, and when most people hear this they assume a reaction occurs. However, you can mix hydrogen and oxygen gas in a balloon and they will do absolutely nothing for eternity. That is, unless you put a match to them. By introducing a flame, you add kinetic energy (motion related to heat) to a few molecules, which suddenly become energetic and react. Once a few molecules react, the energy given off turns around and energizes any remaining molecules to react. The net result is literally an explosion—the energy is released in an instantaneous burst of light, heat, and sound. So, always keep in mind that an energetically favorable reaction may or may not proceed depending upon how fast it occurs.

Cellular Sources of Reactive Oxygen Species

Although there are many potential sources of ROS in the human biochemical system, the importance of a number of them is still a controversial subject. In several cases ROS production can be demonstrated in vitro, but whether these systems contribute significantly to ROS levels in vivo has not been conclusively determined. We will focus on two systems where the evidence for in vivo ROS production is strong and then briefly mention some other sources.

An important part of our immune system are cells called phagocytes which circulate in the bloodstream and literally "eat" other cells. When a phagocyte encounters foreign cells such as bacteria or viruses, they physically engulf the cells and then destroy them chemically. When the foreign cell is engulfed, the phagocyte suddenly increases its consumption of oxygen in an event called an oxidative or respiratory burst.[21] In the oxidative burst, oxygen is converted to superoxide, an ROS, by an enzyme called NADPH oxidase.[22] Another enzyme in the phagocyte called superoxide dismutase (SOD) converts the superoxide to hydrogen peroxide, which is also an ROS. A third enzyme, myeloperoxidase, can combine a chloride ion with hydrogen peroxide to make bleach, ClO^-. Bleach is an ROS too, and together the various ROS attack and chemically degrade the invading cell to the point where it dies. Figure 5.16 shows the process of phagocytosis, while the chemical reactions of phagocytosis are shown in Figure 5.17.

The process of engulfing foreign cells and destroying them is a normal and very good thing; it's essential to combating infection. However, remembering the idea that there can be "too much of a good thing," the ROS produced can get out of hand. Leakage of ROS away from the phagocyte can damage perfectly good cells rather than the intended foreign cell targets. The redness, tenderness, heat, and swelling produced at the site of an infected cut is a response to these chemical attacks as phagocytes swarm to the infected area and release their

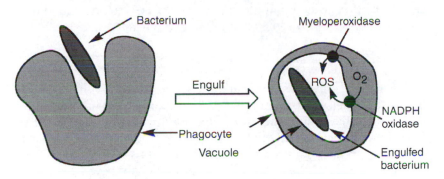

FIGURE 5.16. The process of phagocytosis.

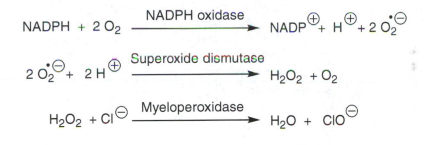

FIGURE 5.17. Reactions employed by phagocytes to destroy engulfed cells.

blast of ROS. It is inevitable that some collateral damage will occur. The fever one experiences with such systemic infections as the flu is also the result of inflammation due to phagocytes releasing ROS.[23]

Another important source of ROS is the digestive process, which, similar to the action of the immune system, is a normal biochemical process. As food is digested, sugar molecules are gradually broken down into smaller molecules.[24] Some of the electrons that were used to form bonds in the sugar molecules are picked up by electron carrier molecules and eventually reach a group of proteins called the electron transport system. This system is located in a structure within the cell called a mitochondrion, and its normal purpose is to capture the energy available from the digestion process. Overall, the reaction causes electrons (tied up in the carrier molecules) to be handed over to oxygen, along with some protons, to make water:

$$4\,e^- + O_2 + 4\,H^+ \rightarrow 2\,H_2O$$

This reaction is the reason that animals breathe oxygen. Although the overall reaction just noted is correct in terms of what molecules go into the process and what molecules come out, this "net" reaction hides the multiple steps along the way. O_2 does not directly react with four electrons and four protons. Instead, electrons are passed through a series of carriers. Only near the end of this chain does oxygen become involved. An enzyme called cytochrome oxidase converts oxygen to water in a multistep process involving three ROS, as shown in Figure 5.18.

It is normal for there to be some leakage of these partly reacted oxygen species from this system, perhaps as much as 2 percent.[25] In fact, as your metabolic rate increases, your oxygen consumption increases, and the amount of ROS that leaks out also increases. Animals kept on a restricted diet live longer than animals allowed to eat what they want. Digesting more food means more oxygen consumption, which in turns means more ROS leakage and damage to various

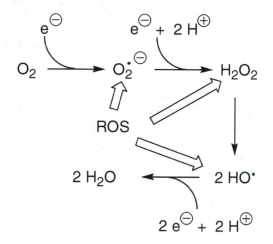

FIGURE 5.18. The conversion of oxygen to water by cytochrome oxidose. Several ROS are produced as intermediates.

molecules, leading apparently to more rapid aging. Furthermore, when you exercise, you are producing more ROS than when you are dozing on the couch. By itself, this is a bad thing, but remember there are other benefits to regular exercise which must be taken into consideration.

There are several other sources of ROS in cells, which I shall briefly mention. When you overdo it exercising, the physical trauma to your muscles damages cells, which then release a number of molecules that can produce ROS. If you are taking drugs, several different systems are activated which destroy foreign molecules. These systems produce ROS in order to degrade the foreign molecule, and leakage can occur from this process too. Finally, lifestyle choices can be a significant source of ROS. Cigarette smoke in particular is a rich source of ROS, which have been invoked as the proximal cause of many smoking-related diseases.

How Do Reactive Oxygen Species Cause Cellular Damage?

Before examining how ROS cause cellular damage, we should briefly think about how to determine when damage has truly occurred. For example, some cells die every day in perfectly healthy people; this is a normal part of life. When they do, the molecules in the cell decay and produce the same molecules as ROS produce when they damage living cells. Thus, any method used to assess the effects of ROS must take into account this baseline level of damaged molecules by the use of appropriate control experiments. Furthermore, in many cases it can be difficult to separate cause and effect. The question of whether inflammation causes the damage or is the result of the damage can be particularly hard to answer. It appears to be a vicious cycle in which a little bit of damage induces inflammation which in turn brings on more damage.

Another circumstance which further complicates studies of the effects of ROS is that our cells have a constant, if low, level of damage occurring all the time. Numerous mechanisms are in place to repair much of that damage. In effect, our bodies operate so that damage and repair are almost balanced most of the time, and normal cellular events cause a rise and fall of our natural defense systems (discussed later in this chapter). As a result, assessing ROS damage by observing changes in the natural defense systems is also tricky. The balance of damage and repair can be upset by illness or disease, and even the normal defense mechanisms, if continually turned on, can create problems. The term *oxidative stress* is usually used to describe the situation in which damage has overrun the repair mechanisms. Much of our knowledge of the role of ROS comes from studying people with certain genetic conditions in which molecular repair systems are defective and thus damage is continually exceeding repair. Ample evidence also suggests that the normal aging process is due to the balance being slightly in favor of excess ROS, so that damaged molecules slowly accumulate in the body.

What exactly is the damage I keep referring to? It is a series of chemical reactions that involve the important molecules that make up a cell. These reactions change the structures and make them unstable or unable to carry out their normal functions. In some cases, the changed molecules themselves cause further problems, but eventually they all end up as damaged goods. It is rather sobering to realize that the types of damage we will consider momentarily are exactly the kind of damage caused by exposure to radiation.[26] The molecules that are damaged are lipids, proteins, and DNA; we'll look at each in turn. Then we will examine a specific disease state to see how damage to particular molecules translates into a significant clinical problem.

LipidDamage

Cell membranes, which provide a selective and protective barrier around cells, are composed of certain kinds of lipids (see Chapter 4 for more on lipids). Direct damage by ROS to the lipids of the cell membrane can be a dangerous problem because the cell may literally fall apart if too many lipids are damaged. However, as we will see in a moment, the damaged molecules create a problem even if the cell does not self-destruct. Lipids and membranes are by far the most thoroughly studied of the various systems that can be damaged by ROS, so we shall spend a bit of time considering how this damage occurs.

Damage to lipids occurs in three stages. The first is known as initiation. In this stage, a primary radical generated by one of the processes described earlier, such as a hydroxyl radical, reacts with a lipid molecule to start things off. Not all lipids are equally reactive, however. The most reactive lipids are those in which a CH_2 group is sandwiched between two double bonds, such as derivatives of linoleic acid and γ-linolenic acid (see Figure 5.19). For example, the hydroxyl radical can pull off one of the CH_2 hydrogens to give water and a new radical species. If we abbreviate the entire lipid as LH, with H understood to specifically represent one of the CH_2 hydrogen atoms between the double bonds, then we can simplify writing the reaction as follows:

$$LH + HO^\bullet \rightarrow H_2O + L^\bullet$$

Once an $L^\bullet$ is formed, things can begin to go crazy in the second stage, called propagation. $L^\bullet$ can react with oxygen, to form $LOO^\bullet$, a peroxyl radical. The peroxyl radical can react with another lipid molecule, removing another H between two double bonds and forming a lipid hydroperoxide (LOOH):

$$L^\bullet + O_2 \rightarrow LOO^\bullet$$
$$LOO^\bullet + LH \rightarrow LOOH + L^\bullet$$

Notice that in each case one of the products of the reaction is the starting material for the other reaction. This is a situation known as a chain reaction, where in principle it is possible for the reactions to go on indefinitely, because they constantly supply more radical species (as long as the supply of lipids and oxygen doesn't run out). One primor-

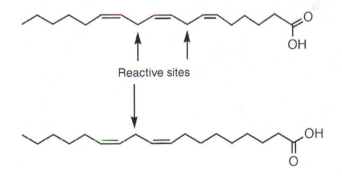

FIGURE 5.19. Reactive sites on unsaturated lipids. Top—γ-linolenic acid; bottom—linoleic acid.

dial, initiating radical can cause the destruction of many lipids because of this multiplying effect. In experimental systems that mimic living cells reasonably closely, about 25 lipids can be destroyed by one primordial radical before the process stops.

As that number indicates, these reactions do not go on forever even if theoretically possible, because eventually one radical encounters another radical, and they annihilate or destroy each other by using their unpaired electrons to form a new covalent bond (similar to the process shown in Figure 3.3). This process is called termination; here are two possible termination reactions:

$$L^\bullet + L^\bullet \rightarrow L–L$$
$$L^\bullet + LOO^\bullet \rightarrow L–OOL$$

Other molecules can also help terminate the chain reaction. We'll address those a little later in this section.[27]

The processes just described can cause destruction of membrane lipids by turning them into lipid hydroperoxides (LOOH), which undergo further reactions. These same processes also cause unsaturated cooking fats to become rancid. As long as oxygen can get to the lipid molecule, this process can occur. The warmer the temperature, the faster the reaction will go, which is why oils used in deep fryers go bad rather quickly. Some preservatives, added to food or packaging, are molecules that are good terminators of radical reactions. For instance, BHT (butylated hydroxy toluene) and BHA (butylated hydroxy anisole), good radical traps (terminators), are incorporated in the paper lining of cereal boxes to prevent the fats in the cereal from going bad.

You may be wondering why converting lipids into lipid hydroperoxides is such a problem, especially since only a relatively small part of the molecule is changed. There are several reasons, but to appreciate them we need to first look at the structure of membranes.

Biological membranes are described as "fluid mosaics" with an underlying organization called a lipid bilayer. This bilayer is composed of lipids such as phosphatidylcholine (described in Chapter 4) and closely related molecules, as well as cholesterol. The important and common characteristic of these lipids and others that participate in membranes is that they have a very polar end (the head), and long, nonpolar tails. When they are placed in water, the "like dissolves like" rule applies. The nonpolar tails associate with each other, while the polar ends orient themselves so that they face the polar water environment. In the case of a cell membrane, the net result is a bilayer, so called because there are two layers of lipids whose nonpolar tails intermingle slightly and whose polar heads face either the exterior or interior of the cell, both of which are aqueous polar environments. Investigations have shown that the lipid bilayer is fluid in the sense that the individual molecules are free to move laterally in the bilayer.[28] As we shall see in a bit, proper fluidity is important to a healthy membrane.

A cell membrane is composed of more than just lipids, and this is reason for the *mosaic* description. A variety of proteins float within the lipid bilayer or are closely associated with the membrane in some way. Some of these proteins are on the outside or inside of the membrane, while others traverse the entire lipid bilayer. The proteins serve several functions. For instance, proteins on the outside of the cell membrane function in cell-cell communication. Proteins that pass all the way through the lipid bilayer may act as receptors, ion channels, or energy generators (we will have more to say about some of these roles in Chapter 6). Overall, the variety of proteins floating and moving laterally in a moving sea of lipid molecules creates the notion of the fluid mosaic (see Figure 5.20).

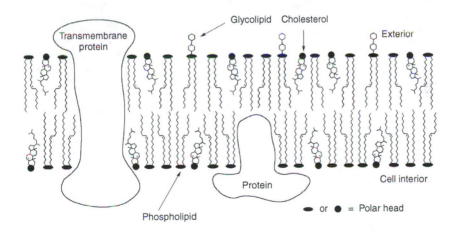

FIGURE 5.20. The fluid mosaic model of a membrane.

As just indicated, properly functioning membranes are fluid, a bit like slightly set gelatin—they are semiliquid. What gives the membrane this fluid characteristic? This fluid state is largely due to how the long lipid tails pack together or, rather, how they don't pack. Molecules that pack together really well are generally very similar in size and shape and tend to form crystals, which are of course solids. Since the membranes are not solid, but not exactly a liquid either, we can conclude that the molecules are not well packed. This comes about for several reasons; I will give the two most important. First, lipid bilayers are made of several different kinds of lipids which have a variety shapes and fatty acid tails. The varying lengths and structures of these tails, as well as the varying types of lipid molecules in general (phosphatidylcholine versus other types, such as cholesterol), prevents them from packing together well. The second reason that membrane lipids do not pack well is that unsaturated lipids in membranes have double bonds with the *cis* geometry (see Figure 5.21). This *cis* arrangement introduces a kink in the tail, which prevents the tails from packing together well, whereas the tails with a *trans* arrangement can all line up in a similar manner. The kink and its effect on shape is clearly visible in Figure 5.20.[29]

With this background we can now return to considering how and why lipid hydroperoxides present a problem. When a lipid in the cell membrane is converted to a lipid hydroperoxide, the normal structure of the membrane is affected in several ways. The hydroperoxide group, –OOH, is introduced into the middle of the nonpolar tail, but –OOH is somewhat polar. This wreaks havoc with the "like dissolves like" rule because the nonpolar tails that were mingling together sud-

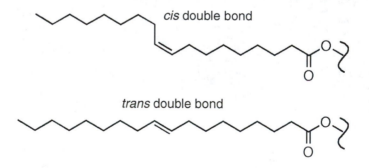

FIGURE 5.21. The effect on shape of *cis* and *trans* double bonds.

denly have a polar group in their midst. If there are a number of lipid hydroperoxides or other forms of damaged lipids present, they tend to congregate together and create regions within the lipid bilayer that are different in fluidity from the rest of the membrane. The result is that some parts of the bilayer become stiffer, similar to more fully set gelatin. Solitary lipid hydroperoxides may push their damaged tails to the polar face of the lipid bilayer to comply with the "like dissolves like" rule. In addition, enzymes called phospholipases exist whose purpose is to remove any fatty acid tails which have been converted to hydroperoxides. If many lipid hydroperoxides have been formed, this enzyme action could remove enough nonpolar tails that the possibility exists for a total failure of the membrane because it is gradually dismantled.

To add insult to injury, the lipid hydroperoxides can undergo a chemical reaction and break apart, forming very reactive and destructive aldehydes. Two things result. First, the broken tail now has a polar end to it, which will not be terribly happy within the nonpolar interior of the membrane. Consequently, it tends to either turn out toward the polar head groups, or it may associate with other damaged lipids and contribute to stiffening of the membrane as described earlier. Second, the reactive aldehyde that is formed can react with proteins embedded in the membrane and cause cross-links between two protein molecules. Such cross-links can also be caused by the lipid hydroperoxides or other ROS acting on the –SH groups of proteins, creating a –S–S– or disulfide bridge between two proteins. Evidence also suggests that the lipids can cross-link with proteins or with themselves. Because of the variety of unsaturated lipids found in membranes, many reactive aldehydes are possible. One well-documented set of reactions is shown in Figure 5.22.

These aldehydes have other insidious effects. They can react directly with a variety of critical enzymes, causing their inhibition. They can react with DNA, which can lead to mutations, and they act as chemotactic substances—molecules which attract other cells. Some of these aldehydes attract phagocytes to the site where they were formed. The phagocytes attack with an oxidative burst, as described earlier, causing more lipid hydroperoxides to be formed. The net result is that the products of the oxidative burst create molecules which attract more cells which create still more damage. I'm sure you can see how this process I've described, which is essentially inflammation, can become self-perpetuating to a degree. Some processes can

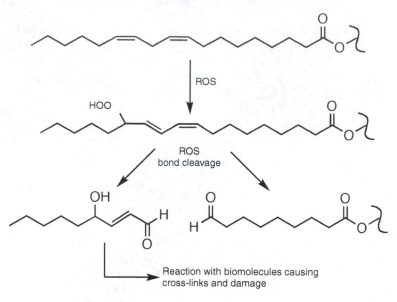

FIGURE 5.22. Reactions of unsaturated lipids leading to reactive aldehydes.

stop the cycle, of course, but it is clear that chronic infections, which keep the phagocytes in constant action, can cause a high level of damage. Evidence suggests that chronic infections are indirectly responsible for about one-third of cancer cases worldwide.

The net result is that both direct damage to the lipids of the bilayer and secondary damage due to cross-linking of various molecules lead to a stiffer membrane. The proper function of membrane proteins requires a fluid membrane because the proteins must be able to change their shape as they do their jobs. Furthermore, processes such as phagocytosis require a flexible membrane. Thus, cross-linking of membrane proteins or damage to the lipids they float in leads to dysfunctional membranes. Data support this model of how ROS affect membranes, and increased membrane stiffness has been demonstrated in aging and several disease states. Figure 5.23 illustrates a damaged membrane with all these effects: damage to lipids, cross-linking of lipids, cross-linking of proteins, formation of such reactive species as hydroperoxides, and changes in membrane structure due to changes in polarity of the chains.

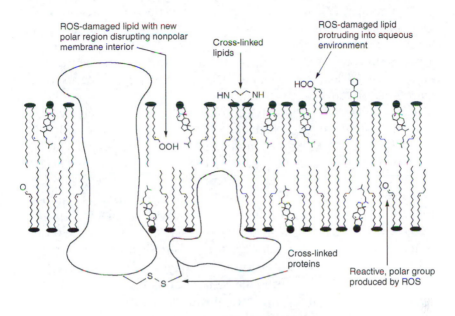

FIGURE 5.23. ROS-damaged membrane.

ProteinDamage

Proteins have much more variety to their structure and function than do lipids, and they are much larger molecules. As a result, they are harder to study, and far fewer investigations of protein oxidative damage have been conducted. However, in recent years more detail has become available on what happens when proteins are damaged. It is clear that damaged proteins accumulate in an age-dependent manner. Damaged proteins are not repaired but instead are chopped up and the atoms recycled by enzymes called proteases. Several studies have shown that protease activity is really too low to remove all the damaged proteins that accumulate over a lifetime. The result is that cells gradually become junkyards for old damaged proteins. The current theory is that at some point the damaged goods interfere with proper functioning of cells. How this might matter is probably most easily visualized by thinking about structural proteins that make up skin, muscle, and ligaments. As these molecules are damaged, their functions, such as giving elasticity and strength, decline.

On a molecular level, protein damage falls into two categories. The first is damage to the protein backbone, the long chain of atoms that forms a framework for the molecule. In this case damage means breaking the backbone, which means the protein is broken into two or more pieces. Clearly, this major damage in nearly all cases would render the protein nonfunctional.

The second category is damage to the side chains, which are the atoms and functional groups attached to the backbone. The sulfhydryl or thiol groups (–SH) of the amino acid cysteine are very sensitive to oxidation in two ways: they can gain oxygen atoms, or two nearby –SH groups can be oxidized to form a disulfide bridge (–S–S–). In many proteins disulfide bridges between different parts of the molecule are part of the normal structure. If, however, the disulfide bridges cannot be formed due to oxidation of the –SH groups, then the protein cannot fold up into its functional form. Furthermore, undesired disulfide bridges between two proteins may be formed. Sulfhydryl groups also associate with metal ions in certain classes of proteins (this is also called *complexing* or *coordinating*). If they become oxidized, they will no longer complex the metal ions, which are essential to the functioning of the protein. Any of these changes to the sulfur functional groups on a protein would significantly alter the properties of the protein.

Other amino acid side chains can be damaged too. In many cases, the damage leads to the formation of a carbonyl group of some kind (C=O). For example, the reactive aldehydes formed from *damaged lipids* can react with some side chains. The side chains of imidazole, lysine, and cysteine fit into this category. Figure 5.24 illustrates some of these pathways for damaging proteins.

Finally, we must keep in mind that proteins are constructed from the information in DNA molecules. Therefore, damage to DNA, discussed in the next section, can lead to incorrectly made proteins. These are better described as abnormal rather than damaged, in the sense that we have been using the term, but the outcome is much the same. Furthermore, damage to proteins that regulate the synthesis of DNA and the transcription of DNA into RNA has even more profound implications. If some of the proteins which normally bind to DNA and turn off growth regulating genes are damaged, one may end up with cells that grow out of control—cancer.

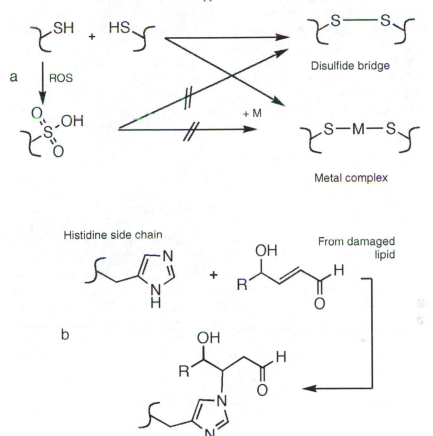

FIGURE 5.24. Mechanisms of protein damage. a: reactions of –SH groups; M = a metal ion; b: effect of reactive aldehydes derived from damaged lipids.

DNADamage

ROS can readily damage DNA molecules. Because DNA is our genetic information, and directs all the operations of the cell, such damage can have a multitude of effects. For instance, damage to the DNA in our reproductive cells can, if not repaired, lead to a mutation which is passed on to the next generation. Some mutations will have no effect, but of course some have dramatic, even fatal effects. But even damage to the DNA in our nonreproductive cells can be serious. A mutation in the DNA changes the sequence of the RNA made from that DNA. Then an incorrect amino acid may be built into the protein, which may prove to be functionally defective. In addition, damage to the DNA that codes for regulatory proteins may result in entire genes that are not "turned on" any longer, which means that some proteins may not be made at all. Alternatively, as described previously under protein damage, some genes may be turned on all the time, resulting in cancer.

One of the best studied forms of damage to DNA is the oxidation of the base guanine to 8-oxoguanine (Figure 5.25). The damaged base is not properly recognized by the DNA-replicating enzymes, and this can lead to permanent mutations. Normally, the G would be paired with a C. However, when 8-oxoG is present, an A is mistakenly installed as its partner. Eventually, with another round of replication, that A is paired with a T. The net result is that a G:C base pair becomes an T:A base pair. The seriousness of such mutations is indicated by the observation that virtually all organisms have elaborate sets of enzymes designed to recognize and remove damaged bases or mispaired bases. Individual organisms which have a defect (mutation) in the genes that code for the repair enzymes are unable to effect the necessary repairs, and this adds insult to injury. People with such mutations generally have a much higher risk of cancer.

Antioxidants and Other Defense Systems

EnzymaticDefenses

The human body contains a number of molecules designed to help prevent ROS damage.[30] These fall into two categories: enzymatic de-

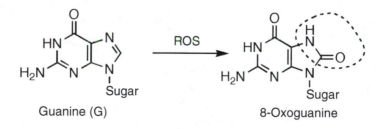

FIGURE 5.25. ROS damage to the DNA base guanine.

fenses and dietary antioxidants. Among the enzymatic defenses are superoxide dismutase (mentioned earlier in connection with the oxidative burst) and an enzyme called catalase. Superoxide dismutase converts superoxide ($O_2^{\bullet-}$) to hydrogen peroxide (H_2O_2), which is still an ROS. Catalase then destroys the hydrogen peroxide. These reactions are shown in Figure 5.26, part a. Superoxide dismutase exists in several different forms, but each requires metal ions to function. This accounts in part for our nutritional need for small amounts of the metals zinc, copper, and manganese.

Another defensive enzymatic system is based upon the molecule glutathione, which is composed of three amino acids linked together into a tripeptide. The business end of glutathione is an –SH group, called a thiol or sulfhydryl. Glutathione is usually abbreviated GSH; it reacts with hydrogen peroxide to form water and a dimer of glutathione. The enzyme that carries out this reaction is called glutathione peroxidase; the glutathione dimer that results (GS–SG, which has a disulfide bridge) can be recycled by another enzyme called glutathione reductase with the aid of NADPH. Glutathione peroxidase requires the metal selenium in trace amounts. Figure 5.26, part b, shows how these molecules work together to destroy H_2O_2.

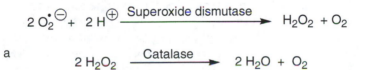

a

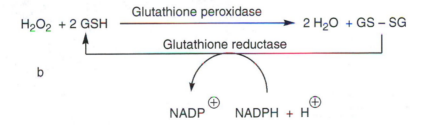

b

FIGURE 5.26. Enzymatic defenses. a: destruction of superoxide; b: the protective role of glutathione, GSH.

Dietary Antioxidants

It is apparent from many studies of humans that the consumption of high levels of fruits and vegetables leads to a lower incidence of such degenerative diseases as cardiovascular problems and cataracts, as well as cancer. A particularly alarming statistic is that people with the lowest fruit and vegetable consumption have about double the rate of cancers of the colon, stomach, esophagus, lung, pancreas, cervix, and ovary, compared to people who consume many fruits and vegetables.[31] Dietary antioxidants appear to be responsible for this difference. Some dietary antioxidants, such as vitamin E, vitamin C, and carotenoids like β-carotene, have been known for a long time to be important diet components with several functions, but their role as antioxidants has only been appreciated more recently. Other dietary antioxidants, such as the flavonoids and related phenolic compounds, have only recently been recognized for their important role.[32] In fact, the evidence suggests that the flavonoids are more important antioxidants than vitamins C or E, or β-carotene. Just about all fruits and vegetables contain antioxidants—that old saying about an apple a day keeping the doctor away is probably truer than anyone realized. The list in Exhibit 5.1 gives some examples of foods that have potent antioxidant properties.[33]

Many people will be heartened to find red wine and dark chocolate on this list. As it turns out, red wine consumption was an important clue about the role of antioxidants in cardiovascular disease, which added greatly to our understanding of this disease. In what has become known as the French paradox, it was discovered that people in a particular region in France who ate a large amount of fat in their diet

EXHIBIT 5.1. Antioxidant-rich foods.

Garlic	Concord grape juice
Kale	Strawberries
Spinach	Red wine
Brussels sprouts	Dark chocolate
Alfalfa sprouts	Green tea
Broccoli flowers	Black tea
Beets	

and therefore should have had a high incidence of cardiovascular disease did not. It was soon ascertained that the flavonoid and phenolic content of the local grapes and the resulting red wine was responsible for the protective effect. Some important antioxidant compounds are shown in Figure 5.27.

Studies of the antioxidant capacity of large numbers of flavonoids and related phenolic compounds show that the most potent flavonoid antioxidants have the core structure shown in Figure 5.27. Studies also indicate that the glycosides of flavonoids are less active than the aglycones. Still other studies have demonstrated that a large portion of flavonoids absorbed in humans are metabolized to phenolic acids (similar to gallic acid), which appear to be equally good as antioxidants.

How exactly do the flavonoids and other dietary antioxidants act to reduce damage by ROS? A good antioxidant is able to react with a ROS by trading a hydrogen atom to give a free radical, but one that is very stable and unreactive (essentially an *un*reactive oxygen species, an "unROS"). The secret lies in their structures. Compounds with a phenolic structure, especially one with two alcohols and an extended ring system, readily give up their hydrogen and become a stable free radical. Several different antioxidants can pass along or trade the extra electron, until it resides in the most stable molecule. For instance, LOO• or L•, two types of radicals formed from damage to a lipid, can react with vitamin E, which has a phenolic group. The free radical formed from vitamin E can then react with a flavonoid. An additional reactive free radical (such as LOO• or L• but other radicals are possible) can react further with the flavonoid radical to eventually give a

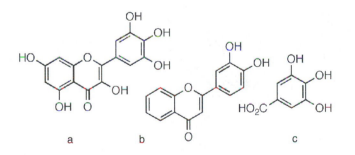

FIGURE 5.27. Dietary antioxidants. a: myricetin, a flavonoid; b: flavonoid structure with the minimal features needed for activity; c: gallic acid, a phenolic acid.

structure which is no longer a free radical. Figure 5.28 shows these pathways; notice that in the scheme vitamin E and the flavonoid are both recycled. NADPH, which is abundant in cells, is ultimately driving this process. The net effect is that any free radical chain reactions, for example, those mentioned in the discussion of lipid damage previously, are terminated because the products of the reaction are unreactive. The more reactive ROS such as the hydroxide radical (HO) can react directly with vitamin E too, and other molecules such as vitamin C or glutathione can play the role of the flavonoid.

Atherosclerosis

Atherosclerosis, more commonly known as hardening of the arteries, is a form of cardiovascular disease. It is a very serious condition that kills many people each year and decreases the quality of life for many more. On a molecular level, atherosclerosis has its origins in ROS damage.

The trouble begins largely with lifestyle choices, although there are genetic aspects as well. A diet high in fat results in high levels of

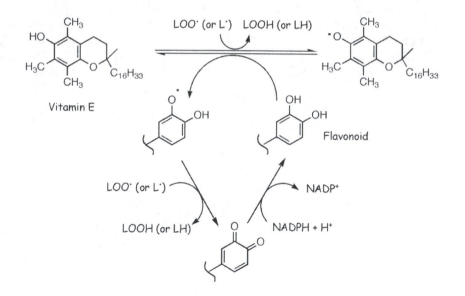

FIGURE 5.28. The role of dietary antioxidants such as flavonoids in quenching or destroying various kinds of ROS.

blood lipids of various kinds. A low intake of dietary antioxidants (as just described) and such habits as smoking increase one's oxidative stress. Infrequent exercise means that the heart is out of condition and pumps less strongly, leading to very slow blood flow, particularly in the capillaries and near branch points in the arteries. These factors and others set the stage for atherosclerosis.

When the blood slows down enough, macrophages (a type of phagocyte) tumble along the walls of the arteries and occasionally stick, and then squeeze in between two endothelial cells (see Figure 5.29). At the same time, particles in the blood referred to as low density lipoproteins (LDL) also occasionally stick and are pulled, along with the macrophages, into the area underneath the first layer of cells. This subendothelial space is where things really begin to go bad. As indicated in earlier sections, oxidative damage is always occurring, and some LDL particles become damaged.[34] In smokers or people low on antioxidant nutrients, the process occurs more frequently. Damaged LDL (marked with an X in Figure 5.29) is attacked with an oxidative burst by the macrophages, as described earlier for phagocytosis. This of course releases more ROS, which can leak and damage even more LDL particles. At the same time, damaged lipids release aldehydes that act as attractants for more macrophages. You can see that a vicious cycle is set up whereby a few damaged molecules are engulfed in a process which creates more damage and calls in more engulfing cells. We hope to keep this process in check by our natural defense systems, but in people with several risk factors the net

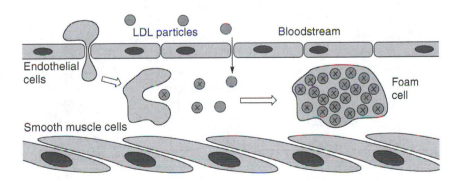

FIGURE 5.29. The process of atherosclerosis.

result is that the subendothelial space gets quite crowded with macrophages. Worse, these macrophages continually munch on the damaged molecules, to the point where they become engorged with damaged LDL particles. These bloated cells are referred to as foam cells due to their appearance under a microscope.

As more foam cells form, they begin to distort the shape of the cells around them. This begins to squeeze the blood vessel closed, and the stage is set for a heart attack if the artery in question is in the heart. Furthermore, the foam cells eventually die because they have too many reactive molecules in them, the result of ROS chopping up the lipids and proteins. As the cells die, their lipid contents are simply deposited in the subendothelial space. In later stages, the smooth muscle cells begin to proliferate and synthesize collagen, the protein which holds our skin together. The collagen is also deposited into the subendothelial space, which becomes a dumping ground for damaged molecules held together by a matrix of collagen. Finally, cholesterol and the calcium salts begin to precipitate as crystals. This is the ultimate "hardened artery," and obviously we'd like to avoid it.

Are there ways to avoid developing atherosclerosis? Certainly. Smoking and avoiding exercise are two great ways to bring atherosclerosis on, as you can see from the description of how the process gets started. Proper nutrition, especially a generous intake of fruits and vegetables which are rich in antioxidants, is important. This is because an LDL particle contains vitamin E in addition to protein and lipids, and a variety of antioxidants can help regenerate the vitamin E after it has taken the initial damage from ROS.

We have now come full circle on the topic of antioxidants, ROS and chemical reactivity. We have seen that a variety of normal processes produce ROS. Our bodies have mechanisms to deal with them, although studies on aging and oxidative stress suggest that our natural defense mechanisms lag slightly behind the ROS load. We have also seen that many situations such as disease produce excess ROS, more than our natural defense systems can handle. The balance between production and destruction of ROS is critical and can be tipped in either direction. Based upon the chemistry discussed, it is clear that long-term consumption of fruits and vegetables can push the balance significantly in favor of the destruction of ROS, to the benefit of our overall health. Because this is a long-term effect and not the treatment of an acute disease, people may not recognize it as a use of medicinal plants, but that is exactly what it is. Appreciation of this fact is growing, with studies on functional foods and nutraceuticals now becoming common. With an understanding of oxidative stress and the chemistry that both causes it and can reduce it, we are poised for much greater discoveries.

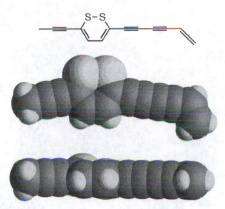

FIGURE 3.20. Thiarubrine A. Top: Lewis structure. Bottom: space-filling views from two perspectives. Atoms are typically colored as follows: carbon—gray; hydrogen—cyan; nitrogen—dark blue; oxygen—red; sulfur—yellow; phosphorous—magenta.

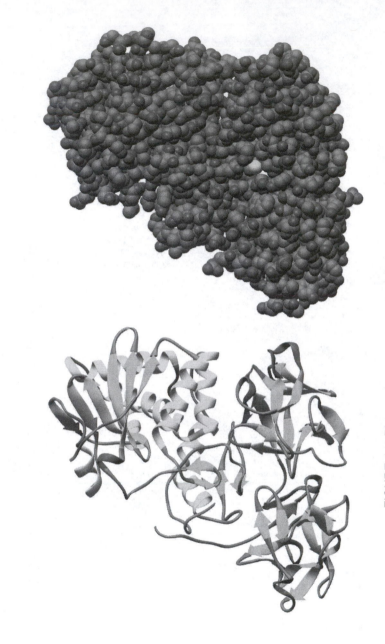

FIGURE 4.7. Ricin. Left: ribbon style model; right: space-filling model.

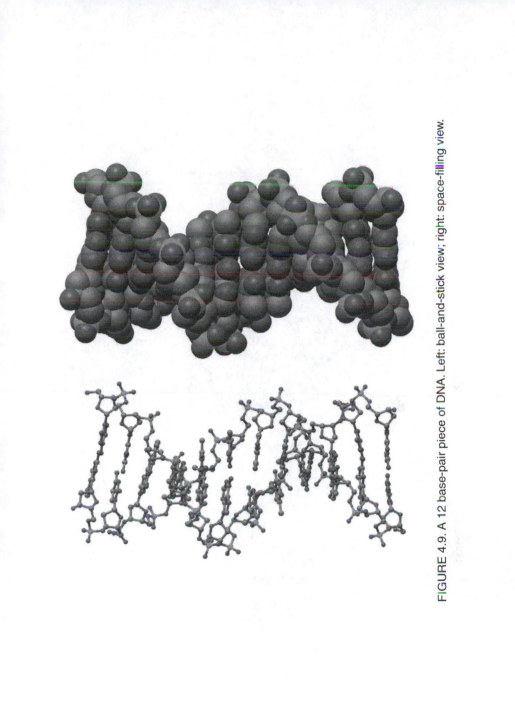

FIGURE 4.9. A 12 base-pair piece of DNA. Left: ball-and-stick view; right: space-filling view.

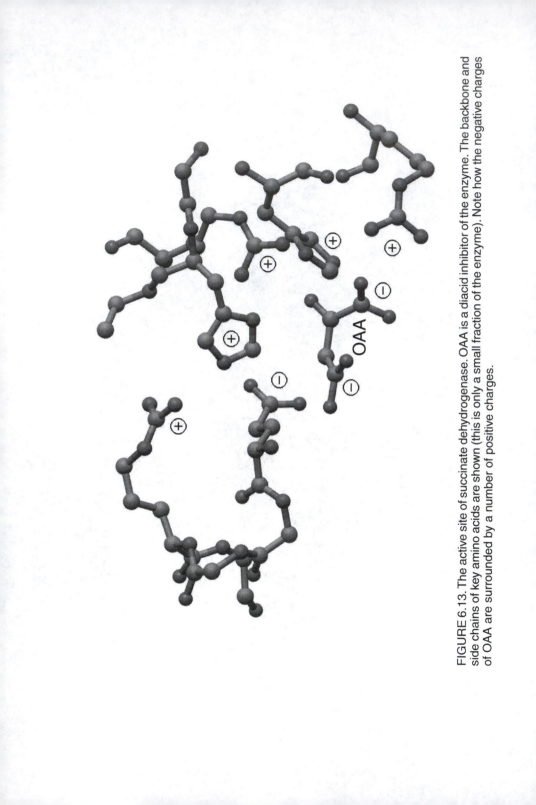

FIGURE 6.13. The active site of succinate dehydrogenase. OAA is a diacid inhibitor of the enzyme. The backbone and side chains of key amino acids are shown (this is only a small fraction of the enzyme). Note how the negative charges of OAA are surrounded by a number of positive charges.

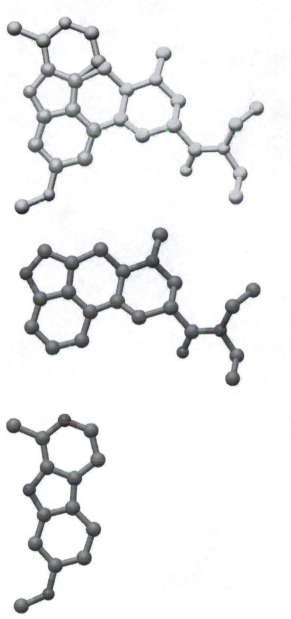

FIGURE 7.7. Comparision of harmine with LSD. Left: Harmine; middle: LSD; right: overlay of the two molecules. In the overlay, harmine is cyan and LSD lavender. The nine gold atoms are common to both molecules and were aligned to overlay the two molecules.

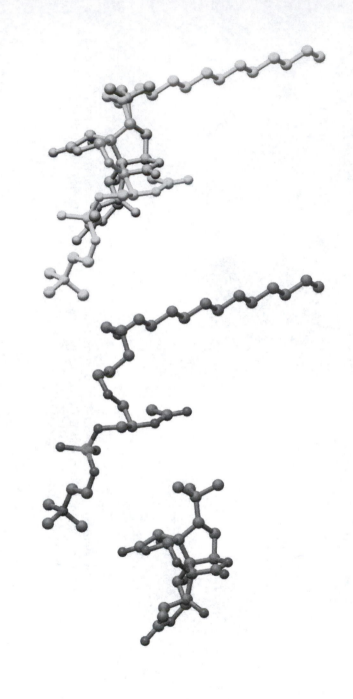

FIGURE 7.10. Comparison of ginkgolide B with PAF. Left: Ginkgolide B; middle: PAF; right: overlay of the two molecules. In the overlay, ginkgolide B is lavender and PAF is cyan. The four gold atoms are common to both molecules and were aligned to overlay the two molecules.

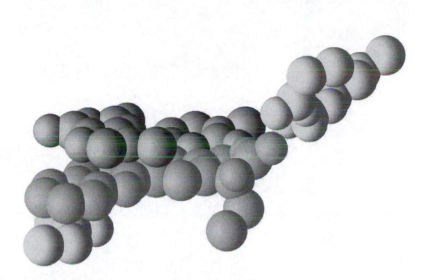

FIGURE 7.16b. Space-filling view of Figure 7.16a. The protein (TOP1) is shown in cyan, the DNA strand in lavender, and camtothecin in gold. Note how the flat camptothecin molecule is sandwiched (intercalated) between a group from TOP1 and one of the DNA bases (the other DNA base is at the rear in the same plane as camptothecin).

Chapter 6

Drug Delivery and Action

Now that we have considered some important background material, the next two chapters address the "meat" of the book: how drugs (and toxins) work in the body. First, we will look at some general principles of pharmacology, the science of drug delivery and action. As we do so we will move again to thinking about individual molecules and how they act on a molecular level. Then, in Chapter 7, we'll use a case study approach to apply all that we have learned to understand how several different plant drugs are believed to work.

DELIVERING DRUG MOLECULES

Before a drug or toxin can have any effect, it must be consumed in some manner and begin to circulate in the blood, eventually reaching the intended cells. However, once in the system, a drug does not remain forever. Many drugs are metabolized (changed chemically), and all are excreted sooner or later. In this first section we will discuss some of the concepts of absorption, distribution, metabolism, and excretion of drugs (abbreviated ADME).

Drug Absorption and Distribution

TakingDrugs"

Drugs can be consumed in a variety of ways. They can be

- inhaled (or smoked) into the lungs (tobacco);
- snorted into the nasal passages (insufflation, technically speaking; cocaine);
- taken orally (various teas);

- absorbed through the skin (including suppositories, aloe); and
- given by injection (derivatives or purified plant drugs).

The same drug given by different routes will often behave very differently. This is because a molecule will encounter different metabolic processes depending upon where it is administered. For example, a drug taken orally is subject to the highly acidic environment of the stomach, which can cause a chemical change (a reaction) to occur. The stomach also contains digestive enzymes and microorganisms that can alter a drug's structure. These structural changes might make a molecule less effective as a drug, or they may activate it to make it more effective. On the other hand, the same drug, given instead by injection, does not encounter these particular processes and so it may have a rather different action. We will discuss these metabolic changes more in just a bit.

Another reason drugs may behave differently when given by different means has to do with how quickly they are absorbed. Drugs taken orally may take some time to pass through the initial barriers and build up to a useful level in the bloodstream. On the other hand, drugs that are snorted are frequently very quickly absorbed via the nasal mucous membranes, and an effect becomes immediately obvious. These differences fall into the area of pharmacokinetics—how fast a drug is absorbed and distributed.[1]

One other aspect of delivery is worth mentioning: the idea of localization of a drug. Some drugs are intended to be circulated throughout the body via the bloodstream, but others are really intended only for certain organs. For instance, treatments for asthma or respiratory infections can be very effective if delivered *only* to the lungs. That way, the drug does not encounter the metabolic processes of the stomach, as it would if it were given orally. Of course, the lungs are the desired site of treatment. Since metabolism frequently destroys a significant fraction of the drug, much more of the drug would have to be given orally to get the same effect in the lungs. With higher dosages comes a greatly increased chance of side effects. Unfortunately, to reach most organs one has to administer the drug to the entire body.

TransportofDrugs

Drugs that are taken orally or by intravenous injection generally end up in the bloodstream where they circulate, and in principle they can reach every organ system and every cell in the body. A few drugs are merely dissolved in the blood, which is mostly water (and therefore polar). The majority of drugs in the bloodstream, however, are bound to proteins that also circulate in the blood. A common example is the protein albumin, which plays a part in the immune system. Quite apart from any immune system functions, many drug molecules will bind or stick to albumin. An equilibrium is set up in which most of the drug is bound to albumin, but a small amount is available free in the bloodstream. Only the free (unbound) drug can move into cells or organs and produce an effect because the albumin/drug complex is too big to pass most membranes, as discussed in the next section.

The idea behind chemical equilibrium is that the proportions of each chemical species in the equation are kept constant. Figure 6.1 shows a typical situation where 90 percent of the drug that is given to the patient is actually bound to albumin, and only 10 percent is available to move into the tissues. Yet each time a free drug molecule moves into a cell, an albumin/drug complex breaks up and provides a new free drug molecule (the equilibrium process is trying to maintain the 9:1 ratio of complexed:free drug). In effect, the albumin/drug complex acts as a drug reservoir and provides a more even level of available drug in the bloodstream. A drug which is bound to albumin also escapes much of the metabolic destruction that the free drug will encounter (see the section later in this chapter on metabolism). Thus, drugs that bind to albumin are longer acting, in addition to being

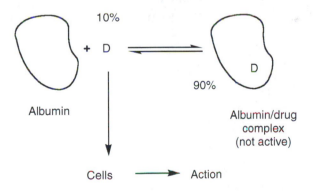

FIGURE 6.1. The binding of a drug to albumin, a protein in the bloodstream, sets up an equilibrium; D = drug.

available at a lower but steady concentration, which reduces the likelihood of side effects.

Binding a drug to a protein confers several advantages as just described. However, it can also cause problems when more one than one drug is taken at a time. For example, if two drugs bind to albumin at the same place, but with very different strengths (affinities), the drug which binds more strongly can displace the drug which binds more weakly. If the weak-binding drug was administered at a typical dose, which assumes, for example, that only 10 percent of the drug is in the free form and readily available to the cells, and the second drug is added, it will release most of the weak-binding drug.

In this case, the free concentration of the weak-binding drug is suddenly much higher than intended, and its desired effects and side effects will be that much greater. Figure 6.2 shows how the system is shifted in the direction of the stronger and more stable complex between albumin and the strong-binding drug. The result is the weak-binding drug is released in its free form to enter the cells at a much higher level. When one hears of "drug interactions" this sort of process is often the cause.

BarrierstoAbsorptionMembranes

Regardless of how a drug is administered, the first barrier it encounters is a membrane. The fluid mosaic model of a membrane was discussed in Chapter 5 and provides a starting point for further consideration of how a drug molecule gets into a cell.

The lipid bilayer of a membrane is composed of two layers of lipids whose nonpolar tails are oriented inward toward each other and

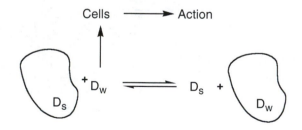

FIGURE 6.2. The competition between a strong-binding (D_s) and weak-binding drug (D_w). If D_w is initially present, and D_s is added, the equilibrium shifts to release more of D_w.

whose polar heads are oriented outward. There they face the polar, aqueous (water) environment of either the interior of the cell or the "outer world." Although the inside and outside surfaces of a lipid bilayer are polar, in terms of size the nonpolar interior of the lipid bilayer is much larger. If a drug molecule is to pass through this membrane and reach the inside of the cell, it must have certain characteristics.

To simply pass (diffuse) through a membrane and into a cell, a drug molecule has to be relatively nonpolar because of the large nonpolar membrane interior (see Figure 6.3). This is somewhat ironic and quite challenging to the medicinal chemist or pharmacologist who tries to design drugs. While a nonpolar molecule can pass through a membrane effectively, nonpolar molecules do not dissolve very well in the aqueous environment of the stomach or the bloodstream. (Remember that water is one of the most polar molecules known; we are using the "like dissolves like" rule here.) Thus, some of the properties needed to make a drug orally available tend to make it cross into cells rather slowly.[2]

The polarity of a drug, and hence its ability to cross a membrane by simple diffusion, is greatly affected by the presence of charge in the molecule. Charge in turn can be affected by the pH of the surroundings. Two functional groups, the amines and the carboxylic acids, can gain or lose a charge depending upon the pH, as shown in Figure 6.4. Although the human intestinal tract begins with the highly acidic stomach, the intestines are more basic as one heads downstream. This

Cell exterior/bloodstream: aqueous, polar

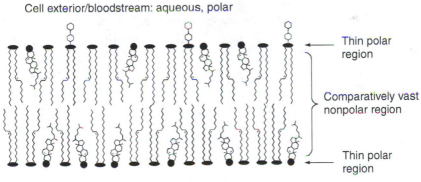

Thin polar region

Comparatively vast nonpolar region

Thin polar region

Cell interior: aqueous, polar

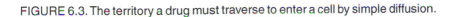

FIGURE 6.3. The territory a drug must traverse to enter a cell by simple diffusion.

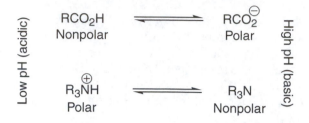

FIGURE 6.4. The effect of pH on charge and therefore on polarity and solubility.

means that the charge on drugs containing an amine or carboxylic acid will vary as they progress through the gastrointestinal system. This variation in charge affects the drug's polarity and therefore its ability to be absorbed will change as it moves through the system.

What I have been describing is the process of simple diffusion across a membrane. Diffusion is the natural action by which molecules spread from areas of high concentration to areas of low concentration. For instance, when a perfume bottle is opened in the corner of a room, the molecules rapidly diffuse out into the room and in short order the fragrance can be detected throughout the room. A drug in high concentration outside a cell, in the bloodstream, tends to diffuse through a cell membrane into the cell where its concentration is lower (provided it has the right polarity, as just discussed).

For some drugs, there are other ways to get across a membrane and into a cell besides simple, passive diffusion. Remember that our model of a membrane is a fluid *mosaic*. The mosaic description refers to the variety of protein molecules that float in the lipid bilayer. Some of the proteins that pass through the entire membrane (called transmembrane proteins) serve as transporters or pumps for certain kinds of naturally occurring molecules. For example, some of the molecules produced during the digestion of sugars must be pumped across membranes in order to be used. Once in a while, one of these transmembrane protein pumps mistakes a drug molecule for the molecule it normally acts on, and the drug molecule is actively but mistakenly pumped into the cell. This is almost impossible to predict in advance, and it can happen to molecules of greatly varying structure and polarity. So although only relatively nonpolar molecules can get into a cell by passive diffusion, any kind of molecule might be accidentally pumped into a cell by one of these transporters.

Finally, it is useful to realize that all membranes are not created equal. On a molecular level, all cell membranes are indeed fluid mosaics. But when you move up to the scale of things as typically seen with a microscope and view several hundred cells at a time surrounding an organ or a capillary, one sees some important differences. When viewed on this larger scale, the blood supply (i.e., capillaries) of some organs are surrounded by cells that form very tight junctions with one another. Other capillaries in different organs have a lining of cells with small gaps between them, which allow molecules in the blood or surrounding (interstitial) fluid to move fairly freely in and out of the organ. Because one of the liver's main roles is to metabolize foreign substances found in the blood, the membranes of liver cells are relatively porous or open. This allows very intimate contact between the substances in the blood and the metabolizing enzymes in the liver. In comparison, the membrane surrounding brain cells is very tight, and very little direct communication occurs between the blood supply of the brain and brain cells. This situation is unique in the body and serves as a protective device for the carefully balanced brain chemistry. The *bloodbrain barrier* is the term given to this tight membrane that makes drug delivery to the brain very difficult, and consequently gives pharmacologists and medicinal chemists much trouble. The differences between tight and open membrane systems are illustrated in Figure 6.5.

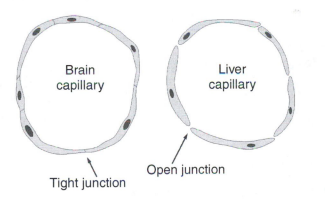

FIGURE 6.5. Open versus tight capillaries.

Drug Metabolism and Elimination

Metabolism

As soon as a drug is in the bloodstream, it begins to be modified by metabolic processes that break it down into smaller pieces or change it in some way. The strategy employed by the human body when it encounters foreign substances, such as drug molecules, is to make them more polar so they can be excreted. The kidney, which is designed to remove small polar molecules from the bloodstream, is the main organ involved in excretion.

The exact means of making molecules more polar depends on the functional groups that are present in the molecule. For examples, drug molecules that contain an ester can be broken down in the blood by enzymes called esterases. When an ester is cleaved, it produces fragments containing an alcohol and a carboxylic acid, both of which are more polar than an ester (and of course they are smaller molecules since the molecules was broken into pieces). Water is a reactant in this process, so this reaction is also referred to as a hydrolysis.[3] This process is illustrated in Figure 6.6 for aspirin, a synthetic molecule that was designed based on a similar molecule found in willow trees. However, the majority of drug metabolism is carried out in the liver, an organ whose main function is the removal of foreign (xenobiotic) molecules. This critical role is one reason why we cannot live without the liver. Unfortunately, long-term exposure to certain foreign substances, such as alcohol in beverages, so overworks the liver that it in effect kills itself. Cirrhosis of the liver from excess alcohol consumption is a well-known example.

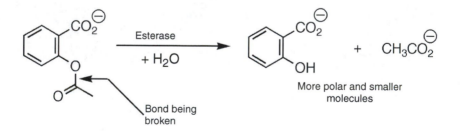

FIGURE 6.6. An esterase adds water to an ester group and creates smaller, more polar molecules.

As discussed previously regarding membrane barriers, the membranes of the liver allow for intimate mixing of molecules in the blood with the liver cells. This is ideal for the blood-cleansing role of the liver, because it allows the enzymes of the liver cells easy access to any foreign molecules in the blood. The metabolic action of the liver toward foreign substances consists of two parts. Phase I metabolism is a series of reactions that alter the structure of molecules, often breaking them into smaller, more polar pieces (similar to what was previously described for esterases in the blood). Phase II metabolism, also called conjugation, is a process in which groups are added to molecules to make them more polar.

In addition to the example of esterases just given, amides can also be hydrolyzed to create more polar molecules. Other examples of Phase I metabolism include oxidative[4] processes such as hydroxylations (adding an –OH group), conversion of alcohol groups to carboxylic acids, and the breakdown of amines to aldehydes or ketones. Note that in all cases, the molecules become more polar. Many other types of chemical reactions also fall under the Phase I metabolic umbrella, but these examples suffice to illustrate the process of making molecules more polar. Each reaction is carried out by an enzyme; some general examples are shown in Figure 6.7.

Phase II metabolism is composed of reactions that make molecules more polar by adding a polar group to the molecule. Two typical ex-

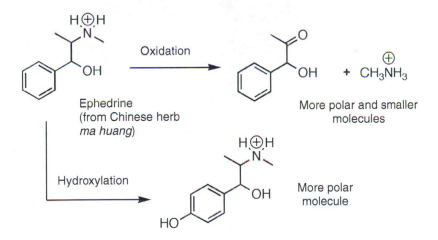

FIGURE 6.7. Additional examples of Phase I metabolism.

amples, illustrated in Figure 6.8, are the addition of glucuronic acid (itself an oxidized sugar derivative) and the addition of a sulfate group. Again, each of these enzyme-mediated transformations make the molecule significantly more polar, and thus more likely to be processed by the kidney and excreted in the urine. As discussed in Chapter 4, many plant molecules, especially those with phenolic hydroxyl groups, exist in the plant as glycosides (combinations with sugar molecules). This makes the molecules more polar and thus more soluble in the aqueous environment of plant cells. The Phase II metabolic process of adding a glucuronic acid residue to a molecule gives a structure reminiscent of the glycosides. When a plant glycoside is ingested, it usually loses its sugar groups in the acid environment of the stomach, leaving the aglycone, which is less polar. Phase II metabolic reactions in which a glucuronic acid is added to a molecule are almost exactly the reverse of this process. The similarities are illustrated in Figure 6.9.

In addition to the reactions involved in these metabolic processes, some other interesting things can happen along the way. One very important enzyme involved in Phase I metabolism, called cytochrome P450 (or CYP), has caused the best-laid pharmaceutical plans to go awry. This enzyme is an oxidase that can add oxygen atoms and functional groups to a molecule (and will act on a wide variety of molecules). It turns out that CYP is an inducible enzyme, which means

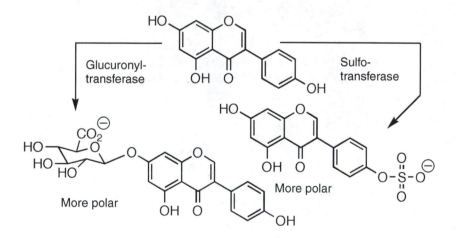

FIGURE 6.8. Phase II metabolic conversions.

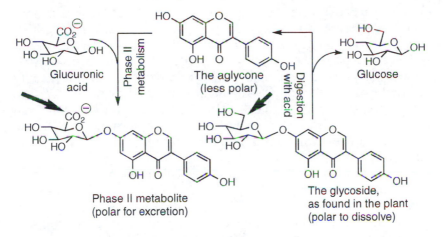

FIGURE 6.9. The parallels between the structures and functions of glycosides and Phase II metabolites. The heavy arrow shows the point of difference.

that if foreign molecules (drugs) are present for a period of time, a signal is sent which causes more of this enzyme to be produced. Thus, if one were taking a drug for 20 days, the amount of drug in your bloodstream would gradually be decreasing even though you are taking the same daily dose. This is because at first only a small amount of CYP is present, but gradually more and more is produced. As more CYP is produced, the drug molecule is metabolized and excreted faster. This is one way that people can build up a resistance to drugs, the situation in which they have to keep increasing the dose to get the same effect. If an individual is taking more than one drug at a time, the effect of CYP may be different for each drug, which can lead to another layer of effects, which can be difficult to decipher. Sometimes this can lead to problems in dosing, but sometimes this induction of CYP is part of how a plant drug exerts its positive effects. For instance, some components of green tea *Camellia sinensis)* have been shown to protect against certain carcinogens by inducing the CYP genes that destroy the carcinogens.

Another twist that CYP adds to drug metabolism is that several closely related types of CYP exist. These are referred to as isozymes.[5] Some isozymes will metabolize certain drugs faster than other isozymes. Since isozymes are enzymes, which are proteins, and proteins are coded for by DNA, people can inherit different isozymes. This is one reason why certain people (fast metabolizers) are less affected by some kinds of drugs than others are. It is also the reason that some ethnic groups are less affected. Because of common ancestry, these groups share genes for specific CYP isozymes. The effect could be just the opposite too: a person or a group could be more sensitive to a drug because the particular CYP isozyme he or she has inherited metabolizes that drug more slowly. As shown in Figure 6.10, these slow metabolizers will require much lower doses of some drugs than other people to acheive the desired effect. If they are given a standard dose, they process it much more slowly, which means the blood level is higher than average. In turn, this means they may have more and perhaps toxic side effects (as well as greater intended effects).

Another important Phase I metabolic enzyme that is found in several isozyme forms is monoamine oxidase (MAO). MAO can metabolize a variety of molecules containing the amine functional group,[6]

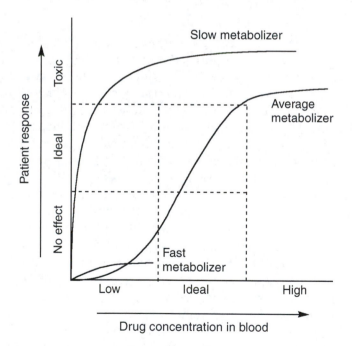

FIGURE 6.10. The effect of inherited metabolic capabilities (isozymes) on the response to a drug.

and, like CYP, some people have more active forms of MAO than others. People's differing response to the Calabar bean as an ordeal poison (discussed in Chapter 4) may be due to their differing MAO isozymes (but it may equally well be due to differences between individual plants, or the season, or what the person ate prior to taking the beans, etc.). The key idea here is that one's inherited genetic material can affect how one responds to certain drugs, based on a change in metabolic rates. Recent advances in biotechnology will permit each of us to determine whether we are a fast or slow metabolizer for many frequently used drugs within just a few years.

EliminationExcretion

Once a molecule has been made more polar, it is the job of the kidneys to filter the drug from the blood and into the urine.

Some drugs, because of their chemical structure, are not well suited to being broken down by Phase I processes or conjugated by Phase II processes. These drugs, which are frequently nonpolar, are still foreign molecules that the body would like to excrete. In these cases, the gallbladder, a small organ intimately associated with the liver, helps out. The gallbladder excretes bile, which is a mixture of nonpolar molecules. Bile can complex with, and dissolve, these nonpolar foreign molecules. Once captured in this way, these compounds are excreted via the feces.

WHERE DRUGS ACT: TARGETS

To exert an effect, a drug must act on a target. The targets that are interesting from a therapeutic view are those molecules and processes which are necessary for the cell to survive, or for an organ to function properly in the context of the entire organism. In broad terms, we can say that a certain organ could be a target. For instance, a drug might act primarily on the brain, or the lungs, or the heart. Organs are typically quite complex and have different types of tissues, structures, and cells within them. So, in narrowing our concept of targets we should realize that at least in principle it would be ideal if a drug could be directed only toward a particular part of the brain, as an example. For instance, the substantia nigra is the part of the brain implicated in

Parkinson's disease, a degenerative disease characterized by tremors in the hands. Likewise, cancers that form tumors can be thought of as a sort of abnormal tissue or organ, and of course cancer is one of the most important targets for drugs.

However, to the scientist, knowing the affected organ or tissue is only the beginning. At the next level of detail, a drug must affect a *process* that occurs in a particular type of cell that is important to the functioning of that cell. Depending upon the nature of the condition to be treated, we might want to turn that process on or off. Examples of processes that various cells must carry out include

- energy production (by breaking down "food"; all cells, all the time);
- cell division (growing cells such as tumors, bone marrow, new tissue);
- neurotransmission (in cells of the central nervous system);
- hormone production (in cells of the endocrine system); and
- motion (e.g., contraction of muscle cells).

Ultimately, the real target is a very specific molecule involved in a particular process within a certain kind of cell. Each of the examples just given can be broken down further into many individual steps. These steps might be chemical reactions involving molecules and enzymes, all of which are potential targets. Some of the steps might also include the binding of one molecule to another (called receptors; this is discussed in the next section), and this binding process is a potential target as well. For instance, a brief description of the process of a nerve signal jumping from one nerve cell to another (neurotransmission) involves the

- synthesis of molecules;
- storage of the molecules;
- release of the molecules in response to an electrical signal;
- binding of the molecules to a receptor on a second nerve cell, and either
- breakdown of the molecules; or
- uptake of the molecules back into the first cell to be reused.

Even these steps have substeps, and in principle each can be a separate target. Clinically, controlling neurotransmission involves such areas as mood alteration, pain control, adjustment of the heart rate, and treatment of asthma. Obviously, the number of potential drug targets is varied and large, and of real importance to human health. In Chapter 7 we will take a case study approach to understanding exactly how some selected plant drugs exert their effect. However, we first return to the molecular level to prepare for the material in the next chapter.

THE MOLECULAR LEVEL OF ACTION

To understand the action of specific drugs derived from medicinal plants, we need to consider the binding of drugs to molecules in the body, as well as explore one more very important aspect of the shapes of molecules.

Receptors, Enzymes, and Binding

Receptors are a class of proteins that have a binding site for a much smaller molecule. The smaller molecule is referred to as a ligand. Generally speaking, receptors are embedded in membranes. When the ligand binds, a signal is sent to the inside of the cell, which in turn causes something else to happen inside the cell. This is the basic means by which different organs and tissues of the human body communicate.[7] Blocking this signal by interfering with ligand binding or turning the signal on by tricking the receptor are important therapeutic strategies. Drugs and toxins obtained from plants are often found to be ligands for medically important receptors, and they have taught us much about the operation of the body. They have also provided a starting point for the design of drugs with desired actions and fewer side effects. Several detailed examples are discussed in Chapter 7.

Enzymes are also proteins, but rather than being involved in signaling processes, enzymes carry out chemical reactions. Any reaction in your body, whether the digestion of food, the copying of DNA, or the growth of new muscle, involves the action of enzymes. The small molecule that an enzyme acts on is usually referred to as a substrate rather than a ligand.[8] Because enzymes are involved in so many bodily functions, they too are important targets for drugs, including those discovered in plants.

Receptors and enzymes recognize their ligands (or substrates) by two basic means: shape and functional groups. You should remember that in Chapter 3 I explained in some depth about the shapes of molecules. We're now in a position to apply that knowledge. In the simplest sense, the shape of a ligand and its receptor must be complementary, like a hand in a glove. In molecular terms, whether a molecule contains a flat system of fused aromatic rings, a long floppy chain of atoms, or a cyclohexane chair, it's these kinds of features that determine its shape. Another aspect of shape is size, and the sizes of the ligand and receptor must also match—a child's hand would fit into an adult glove, but not the other way around, for example. So, a ligand must be of the proper size and have a shape complementary to the binding site of the receptor. Early theorizing about how two molecules could fit together described the situation as a lock and key.[9] However, neither metaphor is complete; we have to consider the functional groups that are present.

Although it may sound strange, a ligand of the right size and shape to fit into a binding site may not actually bind. To bind, the functional groups of the ligand must be oriented to interact with the functional groups on the binding site. These interactions are attractive forces between one functional group and another. The interactions I refer to are derived from the concepts of polarity discussed in Chapter 3, but now we need to be more specific. Three important types of interactions will give us a sufficient conceptual basis to understand some examples.

The strongest of the interactions are the electrostatic attractions between opposite charges, a positive charge attracted to a negative charge. These arise when both receptor and ligand have a charged functional group and they are close enough to attract each other. A hydrogen bond is an intermediate strength attraction.[10] A hydrogen bond occurs when a hydrogen, bonded to an electronegative atom, is attracted to another electronegative atom. This attraction arises from the partial charges on the atoms, which in turn arise from differences in electronegativity (as discussed in Chapter 3). Finally, London forces are very weak forces that attract nonpolar groups to other nonpolar groups. In this context London forces are often called hydrophobic effects, because the nonpolar groups involved "fear" water. Many similarities exist between the notion of hydrophobic effects and the rule given earlier of "like dissolves like." For example, a hydrophobic effect is what causes the long tails of lipids to associate with one another in a membrane (see Figure 5.20). Figure 6.11 gives examples of each of these interactions.[11]

For binding to actually occur, a ligand has to be of the right general shape and the right size and possess functional groups that can be attracted to the functional groups on the receptor or enzyme. The last criterion can be appreciated by modifying the hand-in-glove analogy. To bind, for example, we could say that a certain finger of the hand may require a positive charge on it, so that it can interact with a negative charge on the glove (receptor). The charge would have to be on a particular finger; having it on the thumb or a different finger wouldn't work.

Let's proceed to an actual example, an enzyme called succinate dehydrogenase. This enzyme converts succinate into fumarate (Figure 6.12, part a). This is an important reaction in the conversion of

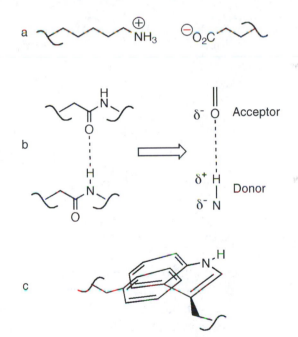

FIGURE 6.11. Examples of attractive forces between functional groups. a: electrostatic attractions; b: hydrogen bonding (indicated by dashed lines); c: hydrophobic attraction (in this case, association of two nonpolar rings).

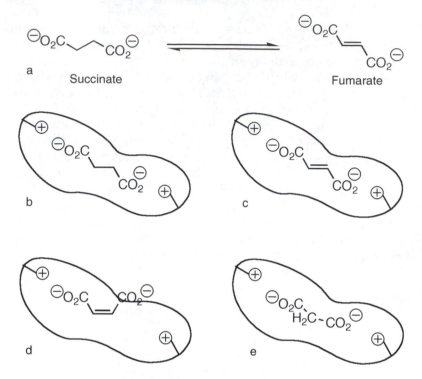

FIGURE 6.12. Succinate dehydrogenase. a: the reaction catalyzed by succinate dehydrogenase; b-e: a schematic depiction of the binding site with various ligands. See text for details.

sugars into energy. Succinate and fumarate are both diacids and possess negative charges in bodily fluids (which are around pH 7.4-7.6[12]). We can hypothesize that the active site[13] on succinate dehydrogenase contains positive charges positioned to attract the negative charges of the diacids (since both succinate and fumarate are part of the reaction, both ought to bind quite well to the active site). Because succinate is composed of flexible single bonds, we can imagine it being oriented in the binding site as shown in Figure 6.12, part b (keep in mind that this is a crude hypothesis and an even cruder diagram). Fumarate, with its *trans,* inflexible double bond, must also be able to fit (see Figure 6.12, part c). We can test our crude model of the active site by looking at how well structurally similar molecules bind to the enzyme. For instance, maleate, the *cis* isomer of fumarate, should not be able to bind very well, as its shape is wrong and it appears that at least part of the molecule would not fit in the active site (see Figure 6.12, part d). Malonate, a diacid which is missing one of the central carbons and therefore can't undergo the reaction, should bind weakly. It fits in the active site, but because of the missing carbon the positive and negative charges are farther from each other and the attractive forces are lessened (see Figure 6.12, part e). We would expect malonate to be an inhibitor[14] of the enzyme because it binds but cannot react.

In reality, experiments have shown that malonate is an excellent inhibitor of succinate dehydrogenase, while maleate inhibits only weakly, consistent with its predicted poor fit in the active site (maleate is about 350 times weaker as an inhibitor than malonate). Experiments that measure the binding strength of small molecules to an enzyme or receptor allow one to speculate about what the binding site must look like, based upon shape and the functional groups present. Often, enough information can be obtained over time to sort out many details and make reasonable predictions about how the binding occurs and how the enzyme or receptor works. Some very powerful techniques can also answer many of these questions in one fell swoop. For instance, X-ray crystallography uses the scattering of X rays from a crystal to give a detailed three-dimensional view of an enzyme or receptor. Such an experiment has been performed with succinate dehydrogenase, and it confirms the scenario just described. Figure 6.13 shows a three-dimensional view of the active site of succinate dehydrogenase (only the portions of the protein backbone and amino acid side chains that are important to binding are shown in the figure). In this case, the active site has an inhibitor called oxaloacetate bound to it (labeled OAA in the figure). Oxaloacetate is also a diacid and a very strong inhibitor of succinate dehydrogenase (about ten times more powerful than malonate as an inhibitor). The figure shows that oxaloacetate is surrounded by at least five positively charged functional groups, consistent with our simple model of the active site. There is also a negative charge nearby which helps stabilize the positive charges.

We could cite many more examples. However, to emphasize the key concept here, it is the shape and size of the molecule that matters, because that in turn positions the various functional groups which

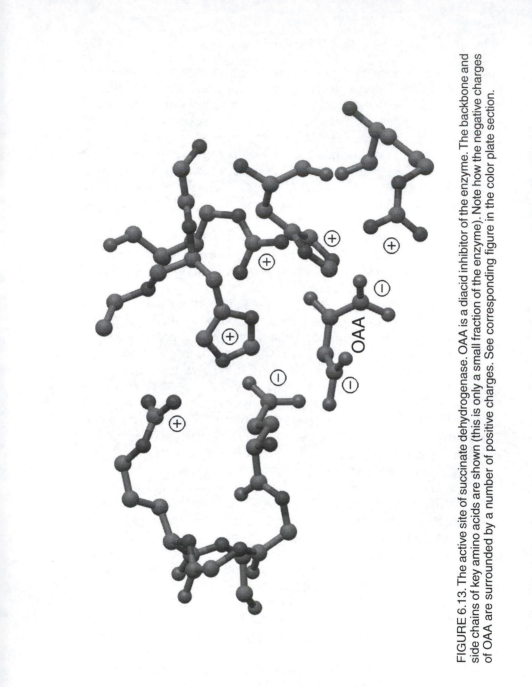

FIGURE 6.13. The active site of succinate dehydrogenase. OAA is a diacid inhibitor of the enzyme. The backbone and side chains of key amino acids are shown (this is only a small fraction of the enzyme). Note how the negative charges of OAA are surrounded by a number of positive charges. See corresponding figure in the color plate section.

contain charges, nonpolar groups, and groups capable of hydrogen-bonding, in the proper orientation to interact with the binding site. This is what makes a substrate bind to the active site of an enzyme, or a ligand to the binding site of a receptor.

A Final Word on the Shapes of Molecules: Chirality

It was no accident that I have been using the analogy of a hand in a glove. One's hands illustrate perfectly our final topic of this chapter: chirality.[15] If you consider your hands or, less conveniently, your feet, you will see that they are similar but not identical. Both hands have four fingers, a thumb, a palm, fingernails, and so forth. But a left hand does not fit into a right-hand glove, so in some way they are not identical. In the chemist's view, we would say that one's hands are a pair of nonsuperimposable mirror images. Everything has a mirror image (except, apparently, vampires), but in many cases the item is identical to its mirror image. A good example would be a coffee mug. One can, in one's imagination, take the mirror image of the mug out of the mirror and superimpose it point for point on the original object. However, the mirror image of your left hand is not your left hand; it's your right hand. Your hands are therefore not superimposable. You can align your palms facing the same way, but then your thumbs are not aligned. If you fix the thumbs, the rest of the hand will not superimpose. Many objects show this property; we say they are chiral. Any item intended for use with your hands or feet is necessarily chiral, but many other objects are as well. For instance, in nature one can find seashells that spiral in a clockwise direction and ones that spiral counterclockwise.

In chemistry the chiral phenomenon appears when a tetrahedral carbon atom has four different groups attached to it. If a tetrahedral carbon atom has two of the attached groups the same and two groups different (see Figure 6.14, part a), then a simple rotation in the molecule makes it possible to superimpose the molecule on its mirror image. On the other hand, if four different groups are surrounding the carbon atom, then no amount of rotation or reorientation will make it possible to superimpose the original molecule on its mirror image. The two are truly different molecules, and they are referred to as a pair of enantiomers (Figure 6.14, part b).[16]

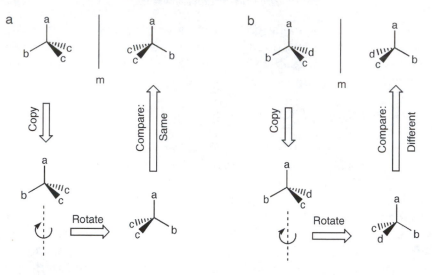

FIGURE 6.14. Chiral and nonchiral molecules. a: an achiral molecule is identical to its mirror image; b: a chiral molecule is not the same as its mirror image; m = mirror plane.

Enzymes and receptors are chiral molecules, and thus they can sense the difference between enantiomers, much as a right-hand glove fits much better on the right hand than on the left. As a result, the issue of chirality affects the medicinal and biological properties of molecules. Figure 6.15 shows two examples of how chirality can make a difference in a molecule's biological behavior. R-carvone is one component of spearmint oil and is largely responsible for its odor. S-carvone, the enantiomer, is found in caraway seeds and triggers an entirely different odor perception. These two molecules smell different to us because the receptors in our nose are themselves chiral and can distinguish between them. The other example in the figure is the molecule albuterol, a synthetic molecule whose structure is similar to ephedrine, a major component of the Chinese herbal medicine ma huang (from the plant *Ephedra sinica;* compare the structure of ephedrine in Figure 6.7 with albuterol). Albuterol is a clinically important bronchodilator used to treat asthma patients when they have acute attacks. Albuterol has a chiral center, and studies have shown that the R isomer is the one with bronchodilating properties; the S isomer is inactive as a bronchodilator but appears to be responsible for cardiovascular side effects in some patients. When it first became

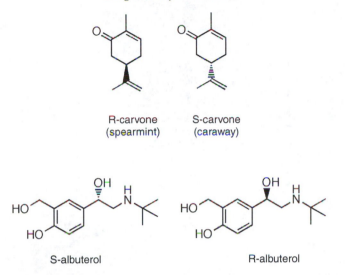

R-carvone
(spearmint)

S-carvone
(caraway)

S-albuterol

R-albuterol

FIGURE 6.15. Enantiomers with different biological activity.

commercially available, the drug was sold as a mixture of both enantiomers.[17] More recently, methods have been developed to make only one enantiomer, rather than the mixture. This can be important to patients because the single enantiomer drug can be taken at a lower dose to get the same response, and it is likely to have fewer side effects because less of it is being taken. It's also important to the pharmaceutical companies, which can patent and market a new drug.[18]

The important point to remember here is that molecules that appear extremely similar, enantiomers, do have different shapes and can have dramatically different biological effects. Almost all molecules found in plants contain chiral centers, and they may be absorbed at different rates, metabolized at different rates, and bind to receptors and enzymes with different affinities.[19] Most of the molecules discussed in the case studies of Chapter 7 have chiral centers, which profoundly affect their action.

SUGGESTED READING

Restak, R. M. (1994). *Receptors*. New York: Bantam Books. Individual chapters discuss different neurotransmitters and drugs that affect brain function.

Chapter 7

Case Studies of Selected Plant Drugs

What is there that is not poison? All things are poison and nothing is without poison. Solely the dose determines that a thing is not a poison.

Paracelsus (1493-1541)

The poisons are our principle medicines, which kill the disease and save the life.

Ralph Waldo Emerson (1803-1882)

Numerous herbal products have reasonably well-documented medicinal activity. In fact, many herbal products have multiple therapeutic effects, which shouldn't surprise us—as we've learned, a variety of chemicals are present in any plant. Unfortunately, relatively few plants have been investigated in great detail. In this chapter we will look at several plants whose biological activity *is* fairly well understood. Some will likely be familiar, and others are not exactly the type of herbs you would plant in your garden or read about in the supermarket checkout aisle. I've tried to choose examples which are diverse in their uses and actions and which illustrate the principles and concepts we have seen in earlier sections. In particular, I want to emphasize the connections between molecular structure and the action of a molecule, so that I leave you with a sense of how one determines the other. At the same time, I want you to have an appreciation of how complex the action of a medicinal plant can be, and to avoid the reductionistic tendencies so dominant in scientific analysis of medicinal plants.

AYAHUASCA AND THE CENTRAL NERVOUS SYSTEM

Western medicine has for many centuries tried to distance itself
from the role of subjective spiritual influences in healing. . . .
Today . . . attitudes are changing. . . . As Western science finally
begins to study and appreciate the practical physical benefits of
psychospiritual practices, indigenous healing practices are becoming not only more comprehensible but also more widely appreciated.

M. J. Plotkin
In Search of the Amazonian Plant Masters
and the Healing Sprit of Ayahuasca,
Shaman's Drum 55 (2000)

Ayahuasca and Its Cultural Setting

Ayahuasca is a complex mixture of plants used by indigenous Amazonian peoples for spirit journeying. The journey is typically taken
by an *ayahuasquero,* a type of shaman, and its traditional purpose is
one of diagnosis and healing. The insights obtained by the *ayahuasquero* during the journey provide the basis for the healing that the
ayahuasquero will attempt. These insights might take the form of visions of particular medicinal plants for use, of communication with
the spirits of plants or dead ancestors, or of spirits that have possessed
the patient. Many Western observers consider ayahuasca to be analogous to a religious sacrament.

Before we go any further, I have to acknowledge my own limita-
tions on this topic. This book is titled *Understanding Medicinal
Plants,* but I have to admit that when it comes to this sort of thing, I
don't fully understand the nature of the experience—but I will tell
you about the pharmacology and try to get at what might be happening on a grander scale. We think about medicinal plants as being capable of curing something, but what is the nature of the cure in this
case? Some say the cure is "psychospiritual" in its nature. Unfortunately, this fascinating phenomenon is almost impossible for many
Westerners, raised on a strict diet of separation of self, spirit, and nature, to comprehend. I am one of those Westerners, I guess. I have
been reading, thinking, and teaching in my classes about ayahuasca
for several years and still feel unable to fully understand what is hap-

pening in this type of healing. Fortunately, others have written eloquently of the ayahuasca experience. I will try to summarize some of the botanical, cultural, and philosophical background before we look at how this mixture functions on a molecular level.

As mentioned, ayahuasca is a complex mixture of plants. Two plants are primarily responsible for the psychoactivity: the bark of the liana (vine), *Banisteriopsis caapi,* and the leaves of a shrub, *Psychotria viridis.* However, as many as twenty plants may go into the mixture, and the additional plants appear to modify the psychoactive experience in ways that are not well understood. By the way, ayahuasca means "vine of the soul" or "vine of the dead" in the Quechua tongue; other names for the mixture are yagé, caapi, or la purga (because of the purging nature of ayahuasca).

A name such as vine of the soul or vine of the dead gives you a clue as to what the experience of taking ayahuasca might be like. People describe the ayahuasca experience as full of realistic but wildly colored hallucinations, as a "dissolving" of ego or self, as a means of accessing the sacred dimensions of nature and reality. Indigenous Amazonians report seeing brightly colored large snakes, jaguars, and spirits. Many of these experiences are very positive, leading to feelings of harmony with nature and others, and lasting spiritual clarity. The experience can also be very frightening; people experience death, see demons, or are eaten by snakes, although even these frightening experiences are generally considered to be enlightening. To some, these hallucinations may seem to have something in common with the drug culture of the 1960s. Equating ayahuasca with recreational drug use is not appropriate, however, especially as it is traditionally used.[1]

In fact, ayahuasca is an integral part of traditional Amazonian folk medicine and should be respected as such. Its traditional use takes place in a communal ritual setting under the strict guidance of the *ayahuasquero,* who whistles and sings special songs called *icaros* that help guide the experience. Remember, the purpose is one of healing, rather than merely tripping for personal gratification. In Amazonian cultures, as in most traditional cultures, disease is believed to have a variety of origins including supernatural and psychological sources, as well as sources more eagerly embraced by Western science and medicine (infectious agents, inherited disorders, etc.). The *ayahuasquero* is part doctor, part therapist, part priest, and the ap-

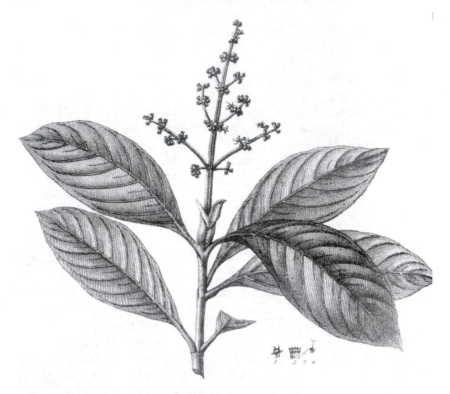

Psychotria viridis. (*Source:* Ruiz, Hipólito. *Flora Peruviana, et Chilensis* sive, Descriptiones, et icones plantarum peruvanarum, et chilensium, secundum systema Linnaeanum digestae, cum characteribus plurium generum evulgatorum reformatis. Lehre: J. Cramer, 1965. Originally published Madrid: G. de Sancha, 1798. Vol. 2, pl. no. 210.)

proach to healing is holistic—the different facets interact and are all important. Keep in mind two things: often, the patient doesn't take the mixture at all, only the doctor, and the mixture usually causes violent vomiting about an hour after ingestion.

Having said this, it is also important to keep in mind that the use of ayahuasca varies and is constantly changing.[2] The traditional, historic rituals certainly varied somewhat from tribe to tribe. But, as the Western world has penetrated into the jungle and people have become more mobile, ayahuasca traditions have changed and been adapted for a more modern lifestyle. Jungle groups that were (perhaps) once relatively ethnically pure have intermarried and moved to the river's edge and then to the city. As is always the case, cultures in contact influence one another. This is readily seen in the use of ayahuasca among mestizo peoples, where it is called *vegetalismo*. In urban Brazil several established churches practice a blend of Catholic and Protestant rituals, and employ ayahuasca as a sacrament of enlightenment. In some cases, these churches have followers in the United States, and as mentioned in note 1 in this chapter, a steady stream of "ayahuasca tourists" journey to the Amazon for the experience.

Finally, I should mention the role of "set and setting" in the experience of psychoactive (or psychedelic[3]) drugs. Set and setting is a phrase made famous by the Harvard psychologist Timothy Leary who experimented with a variety of psychoactive drugs from the 1950s onward. "Set" refers to a person's intentions, expectations, and motivations for taking the drug. "Setting" refers to the physical surroundings as well as the support and guidance of others. A somewhat superficial illustration of set and setting might be the enjoyment of food: eating a relaxed dinner with friends in the atmosphere of an authentic Mexican restaurant is rather different from stuffing a taco in your mouth as you leave the local drive-through restaurant. Investigations have shown that what an individual experiences with one of these drugs is in part dependent upon the cultural context, attitudes, and personality which that particular person brings to the session. Thus, a stockbroker raised in an urban setting may have a very different set of visions than a jungle dweller, although each may still experience something euphoric or frightening. Raves (parties dominated by loud, percussive music, dancing, and the use of the drug Ecstasy) are yet another example of how set and setting play off each other to create a unique experience.

Ayahuasca and other powerful psychoactive drugs cause our brains to experience a reality different than our senses would normally detect, and somehow the set and setting are integrated into that alternative reality. The role of the *ayhuasquero* is to control the setting as the ayahuasca is experienced. Perhaps the *molecules* in ayahuasca are capable of being recreational drugs in a different cultural situation, but they are surely something else in the context of traditional Amazonian societies.

With this background in place, we now turn to the central nervous system, where ayahuasca and many, many other plant drugs exert their influence.

The Nervous System

The human nervous system is exceptionally complex and naturally quite important to our functioning (and our very being, since our consciousness resides in our brains). If asked, most people could state that the central nervous system (CNS) is composed of the brain and spinal cord. Although true, this answer fails to remind us that the nerves leaving the spinal cord and traveling to specific organs are also an important part of the nervous system. In fact, much of modern drug therapy is really therapy of the nervous system, even if the patient doesn't realize it. For instance, if you have trouble with asthma, you probably view this as a lung disease. However, most drugs given in the treatment of asthma are actually affecting the *nerve endings* within the lungs, so a lung problem is really being treated via the nervous system. The same is true for many drug therapies of the cardiovascular system (the heart, veins, and arteries), as well as therapies for excess stomach acid, for example. Generally, all internal organs are controlled to one degree or another by the CNS and its extensions. Given that significance, it is not surprising that the CNS has received the lion's share of research by pharmacologists.

A big part of the complexity of the CNS stems from its anatomy. The brain has many different structures within it, each with particular functions that are often only loosely understood. These structures appear differently under a microscope and generally behave differently in response to chemicals, such as naturally occurring substances or drugs given for a therapeutic purpose. Although difficult to sort out, this complexity is ultimately a good thing because it implies that we might be able to control the various parts independent of one another (in terms of our earlier discussion, structurally different sites controlled by different molecules represent different, useful drug *targets*). Nerves outside the brain also differ from those in the brain, and from each other, in their microscopic anatomy and their chemistry, as do the places where the nerves are ultimately attached to a muscle or organ. Finally, as if things weren't complicated enough, the nervous system also connects to organs which are actually endocrine or hormonal glands (such as your adrenal gland, which supplies adrenaline). Action within the nervous system can lead to release of hormones which in turn affect the performance of organs. Although the endocrine system and the nervous system interact, much of the endocrine system is designed for long-term regulation of bodily function, while the nervous system is devoted largely to more immediate responses.

One of science's ways of coping with complexity is to classify or categorize observations and information, and scientists have done just that with the CNS. The first big division is between the voluntary and involuntary parts of the system. As the names imply, there are parts we can control and parts we cannot. Most of us can make ourselves walk, but we cannot make our hearts stop. The involuntary parts, which turn out to be of greater therapeutic interest, are then divided into two groups, the sympathetic and parasympathetic systems. These categories are shown in Figure 7.1.

The sympathetic system is most easily appreciated as the part that reacts when you are suddenly frightened. All of your body systems prepare for either "fight or flight," as the saying goes. The capacity of your heart and lungs increases in order to supply your muscles with needed oxygen, while other systems ramp up to release muscle fuel

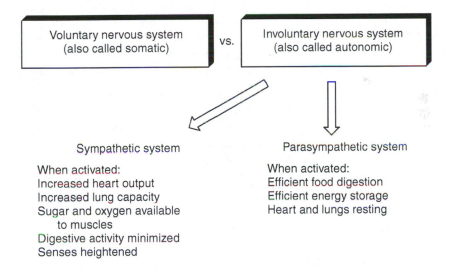

FIGURE 7.1. Classifications of the nervous system.

(glucose and fatty acids). Your senses such as vision and hearing are heightened, and your reaction time decreases. In contrast, the para-sympathetic system kicks in after a meal, and functions to efficiently digest food and store the energy produced. This is a time of bodily rest and repair (think of how you feel after a heavy meal). Although in many ways these two systems may appear to be opposite in function, this is not entirely the case.

Let us turn now to exactly how a nerve impulse travels, because understanding this will give us clues about how we can alter the func-tioning of the system. Nerve cells, known as neurons, carry impulses in an *electrical* fashion along their length. However, what interests us right now is what happens at the junctions between two nerve cells or between a nerve cell and an organ or muscle.

These junctions are known as synapses. In a synapse, transmission of the nerve impulse occurs via *chemical* means. The chemicals that accomplish this are called neurotransmitters. The basic structure of a synapse is deceptively simple; it is a narrow gap between two nerve cells. However, the overall transmission and regulation of the impulse turns out to be very complex. We'll stick to the basics in what follows.

A simple sketch of a synapse is shown in Figure 7.2. Let's follow the nerve impulse as it is travels down the first neuron (at the top of the diagram) toward the synapse. At this point, it exists as an electri-cal signal (you might think of it as an electric current flowing through the cell membrane).

When the electrical signal reaches the synapse, it causes a com-partment filled with neurotransmitter molecules to fuse or join with the cell membrane. The neurotransmitter, shown in the diagram as a black triangle, is released into the synapse (gap) when the container (called a vesicle) fuses or joins with the cell membrane. The synapse is very, very narrow, and the neurotransmitter diffuses across it quite readily. Eventually, the neurotransmitter finds its receptor on the downstream neuron and binds to it. Once the neurotransmitter binds, the receptor, which in our illustration is a type called an ion channel, opens and allows ions to flow into the second neuron (shown by a dot-ted arrow). This flow of ions through the cell membrane starts the electrical signal in the second neuron (remember that ions are charged, so flow of ions equals flow of electricity). The nerve impulse thus continues on to its destination.

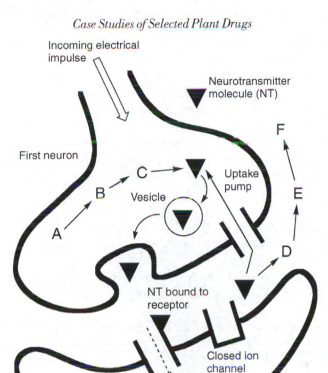

FIGURE 7.2. A simplified synapse. See text for explanation.

Numerous diseases or conditions occur in which this chemical neurotransmission process does not occur properly—it is out of balance somehow. Parkinson's disease is a good example in which activity at certain kinds of synapses is too high, leading to overstimulation of muscle action and thus the shaking or tremors typical of this disease. The complete cause of Parkinson's is more complicated than this, but my brief description illustrates how problems at the synapse lead to clinical symptoms.

When pharmacologists look at this neurotransmission process, they see many ways to control it and potentially do something therapeutic. For example, drugs could be sought that prevent the vesicle from fusing with the cell membrane and releasing the neurotransmitter. Or a drug could be found that blocks the receptor from binding the neurotransmitter, and thus the ion channel won't open. Either of these actions would have the effect of reducing nerve impulse continuation. The first example works by decreasing the amount of neurotransmitter released and thus available to the receptors on the downstream neuron. The second example works by locking the ion channel closed.

These two examples illustrate the major strategies one can employ to alter the workings of a synapse:

- Alter the amount of neurotransmitter
- Alter the behavior of the receptors

The second strategy is a bit less complicated.[4] One who is lucky enough to find drugs that simply lock the ion channel either open or closed has indeed found something useful which allows controls of the nerve impulse.

On the other hand, altering the amount of neurotransmitter in the gap, and thus available to the receptors, is trickier (and consequently more "target rich" in that there are more steps to attempt to control). In the upstream neuron, the neurotransmitter must be synthesized from smaller molecules ($A \rightarrow B \rightarrow C \rightarrow \blacktriangledown$ in the diagram). Each of these steps is carried out by an enzyme; if one of those enzymes can be inhibited (blocked) then we can reduce the amount of neurotransmitter produced. Once synthesized, the neurotransmitter must be pumped into the vesicle, and this is another process that can potentially be inhibited. Finally, the fusion of the vesicle with the cell membrane already mentioned is another target. All of these strategies would serve to reduce the amount of available neurotransmitter and thus tend to stop the nerve impulse.

You may be wondering if there is a way to *increase* the amount of neurotransmitter, and indeed there is. Neurotransmitter molecules do not live forever; they are constantly being broken down and their atoms recycled. This process ($\blacktriangledown \rightarrow D \rightarrow E \rightarrow F$ in the diagram), like the synthesis of the neurotransmitter, is under the control of enzymes which can be inhibited. If you discovered an inhibitor for the enzyme that converts E → F, then the system would back up like a clogged pipe. First, there would be more E because it is not being broken down, then more D, and then more neurotransmitter. More neurotransmitter would in turn mean more open ion channels and more nerve impulses continuing on to their destination.

A final target to consider is referred to as the uptake or reuptake process. Neurotransmitter molecules have multiple destinies—as just mentioned, some are chopped up by enzymes. However, more of them get pumped (or transported) back into the upstream neuron to be repackaged into vesicles and used again (in other words, the whole molecule is reused). If you block the uptake process, then neurotransmitter molecules remain in the gap where they can bind to receptors and continue to cause firing of the downstream neuron. The common mood-altering drug Prozac (fluoxetine) operates this way.

By the way, please don't get the idea that finding all of these drugs that block, inhibit, or do something else interesting is an easy process. Drug discovery is an immensely difficult, expensive, and lengthy process. Many promising drug candidates that do exactly what we want them to do in a test tube are ultimately rejected because they have unacceptable side effects or can't get past the blood brain barrier (recall our earlier discussion of the importance of membranes in Chapter 6). The strategies just discussed for controlling what happens at a synapse are rather theoretical. Actually finding a drug "from scratch" that proves to be useful in people is a different matter. In fact, plants have long provided useful molecules that act on on the synapse. Plant drugs such as ephedra, physostigmine, tubocurarine, cocaine, and reserpine, discussed elsewhere, are good examples.

Before we move on, we should unmask this mysterious neurotransmitter that we keep mentioning. Actually, many neurotransmitters are known, and this is one reason for the complexity of the nervous system. In fact, a single organ is usually controlled by multiple neurons using different neurotransmitters (and don't even ask about the brain!). This creates quite a task for those trying to figure out how these things work, but the multiple points of control do permit our bodies to react flexibly and to respond to a variety of conditions. All of the neurotransmitters are modest-sized molecules. Following are the names of the main ones, in case you run into them:

- GABA (gamma aminobutryic acid)
- Glycine
- Dopamine
- Epinephrine (adrenaline)
- Glutamate
- Acetylcholine
- Serotonin
- Norepineprhine
- Histamine

Each neurotransmitter can interact with a number of receptors; the exact type depends upon the neurotransmitter and the anatomical location.

The Molecules of Ayahuasca

As mentioned at the beginning of this section, ayahuasca contains two main "active" plants: *Banisteriopsis caapi (B. caapi)* and *Psychotria viridis (P. viridis)*. Each of these plays an important role in producing the visions characteristic of the ayahuasca experience by acting on the CNS.

Banisteriopsis caapi contains three major alkaloids that are important in the action of ayahuasca; these are shown in Figure 7.3. These three structures are closely related as they are based on the same ring structure (the β-carboline ring system). They differ only in the number of hydrogens in the right-hand ring (note that tetrahydroharmine

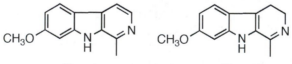

Harmine   Harmaline

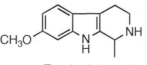

Tetrahydroharmine

FIGURE 7.3. Alkaloids of the carboline family.

has four more hydrogens than harmine, hence the "tetrahydro" prefix). These molecules are slightly psychoactive by themselves, but not enough of them are present in the ayahuasca drink to cause hallucinations. Research has shown that they play an entirely different role in the ayahuasca mixture: they prevent the destruction of a different psychoactive molecule which comes from *P.viridis* .

How is this possible? The ayahuasca preparation is a tea which is drunk, so it is absorbed through the lining of the stomach. Once it passes through the layer of cells designed to absorb and digest nutrients, the molecules in ayahuasca move into the circulatory system and reach the brain, where the real action begins. However, the barrier cells between the stomach and circulatory system contain enzymes designed to help with digestion (and to protect the CNS from external substances that might alter its function). One of these enzymes is monoamine oxidase (MAO). We met MAO earlier when we covered the metabolism of drugs in Chapter 6. Its function is to oxidize (add oxygen to) molecules containing the amine functional group. This is one way of breaking down a molecule into smaller parts for either excretion or recycling by using the parts to build other molecules.

The other molecule, which is found in *P.viridis,* turns out to be an amine as well, so the cells in the stomach would normally digest it by using their MAO enzymes (into a nonpsychoactive substance, as it turns out). However, the role of harmine and its close relatives is to inhibit the digestive action of MAO. By blocking the digestive and oxidative action of MAO, these molecules prevent the breakdown of dimethyltryptamine, which is the psychoactive molecule from *P. viridis* (see Figure 7.4).

Dimethyltryptamine (DMT) is powerfully psychoactive, but it cannot normally be taken orally (as in ayahuasca) due to the action of MAO in the stomach. However, when harmine or its relatives are present, DMT avoids digestion and enters the circulation. Thus, both

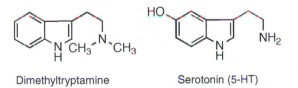

Dimethyltryptamine   Serotonin (5-HT)

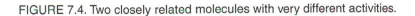

FIGURE 7.4. Two closely related molecules with very different activities.

plant species are essential to a proper ayahuasca mixture. Interestingly, other Amazonian groups use the resin of plants from the genus *Virola,* which also contain DMT, to make a hallucinogenic snuff called ebena. However, because they snort this plant powder, and the DMT is absorbed through the nasal mucous membranes, MAO inhibitors are not needed to produce the desired effect.

The Connection Between DMT and Hallucinations

With this background on the role played by the different molecules in ayahuasca, we can now turn to how DMT causes hallucinations. As is often the case, we have only a partial answer even though many pieces of data are available. DMT is structurally related to the neurotransmitter serotonin, which is also called 5-hydroxytryptamine (and often abbreviated 5-HT; see Figure 7.4).

Serotonin controls many functions of the CNS; the big picture is fairly poorly understood. Some very specific parts of the brain employ serotonin as their chief neurotransmitter, but it is found in virtually all parts of the CNS, and even outside of the CNS. More than a dozen different types of receptors that respond to serotonin in different ways have been identified in recent years, and the classification of receptors is constantly changing. With this kind of complexity on a molecular level, it is not surprising that a variety of conditions have been linked to problems with serotonin functioning:

- Anxiety
- Eating disorders
- Migraines
- Sexual disorders
- Sleep disorders
- Schizophrenia
- Obsessive-compulsive disorder
- Substance abuse

Obviously, proper functioning of the serotonin system is important to the entire human condition—sleep, mood, personality, sex, and cravings are all affected.

Many of our clues about how a serotonin-driven neuron works come from studies using naturally occurring hallucinogenic molecules. A few of these are listed in Table 7.1. Although not all of these

TABLE 7.1. Hallucinogenic molecules and their sources.

Molecule	Source
LSD (lysergic acid diethylamide)	*Claviceps purpurea* (a fungus)
Psilocybin	*Psilocybe mexicana* (a mushroom)
N,N-dimethyl-5-methoxytryptamine	*Bufo alvarius* venom (a toad)[a]
Mescaline	*Lophophora williamsii* (the peyote cactus)

[a]Yes, you read this right. This toad is apparently the only hallucinogenic animal known. For the full story on what toad to use and why you have to smoke the venom, see the article by Andrew Weil and Wade Davis (1994) *Bufo alvarius:* A potent hallucinogen of animal origin. *Journal of Ethnopharmacology,* 41: 1-8.

molecules are found in plants, they have proven useful in understanding DMT and the serotonin system.

What do these molecules have in common that might explain their psychoactivity? If one compares the structures of LSD and psilocybin with the β-carboline alkaloids mentioned earlier, and to DMT and serotonin, a similarity is apparent which might help us decipher how all of them work (remember that the major role of the β-carboline alkaloids in ayahuasca is inhibition of MAO, but they are also mildly hallucinogenic, and thus useful in this analysis). What we would like to do is to develop a hypothesis about which structural similarities are important for psychoactivity. Figure 7.5 shows these molecules with their "common core structure" shown with bold bonds within each of the molecules (although I have not shown the structure of N,N-dimethyl-5-methoxytryptamine, it too follows this pattern). Among these molecules, the common core, which one might hypothesize is responsible for the psychoactivity, contains the indole ring system and a –C–C–N– chain attached to the indole 3 position (or you might say that the molecule tryptamine is embedded within their structures). Although not required for psychoactivity, there is also a "subpattern" in that many of the molecules have an oxygen-containing functional group at position 4, 5, or 6 of the indole ring.

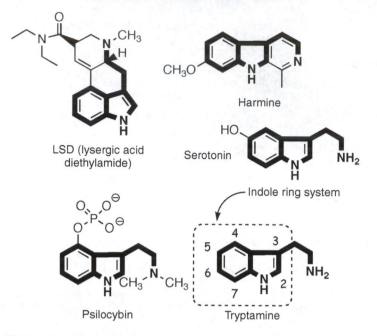

LSD (lysergic acid
diethylamide)

Harmine

Serotonin

Indole ring system

Psilocybin

Tryptamine

FIGURE 7.5. Structural similarity of several neuroactive molecules. The common structure is shown in bold.

You may have noticed that I left mescaline out of Figure 7.5. Mescaline and its many psychoactive, synthetic relatives do not have the same common core structure as the other molecules. If you compare the structure of mescaline with the structure of LSD, you can see a *different* common core structure, which we could describe as an aromatic or benzene ring with a –C–C–N– chain attached (see Figure 7.6). When one takes into account the many synthetic relatives of mescaline, it becomes clear that oxygen-containing functional groups turn out to affect psychoactivity in this series of molecules too.

So altogether we see that among these various psychoactive molecules found in nature, two structural patterns are closely related. Both have the –C–C–N– chain, but in one case it is attached to an indole ring, and in the other it is attached to an aromatic (benzene) ring. Both patterns can be seen embedded within the structure of LSD in slightly different ways, so we may get the most insight from studying LSD (and it is by far the most potent hallucinogen known).

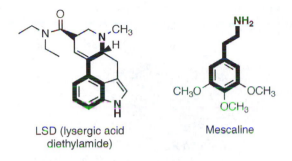

LSD (lysergic acid
diethylamide)

Mescaline

FIGURE 7.6. Structural similarities between LSD and mescaline.

What I have been discussing here is referred to in the pharmaceutical industry as structure-activity relationships (SAR). Patterns such as these are of great interest to medicinal chemists and pharmacologists because they suggest a minimum set of structural features which seem to be required for a particular biological activity. Having provided some starting clues, these natural molecules then inspire the preparation of synthetic drugs. By making a number of synthetic drugs in which the structure varies only a little, medicinal chemists can further define and refine the part of the structure responsible for activity. One general goal when developing any drug is to design a molecule that has the desired effect and very minimal side effects by tweaking the structure. In addition, it should be easy to synthesize (unless the naturally occurring molecule proves to be the most potent).

The information gained from identifying the active core structure can teach us something about how these molecules bind to and activate a receptor. However, the patterns noted are basically those of connectivity—a pattern of rings and chains and particular atoms connected in a certain fashion. As discussed in Chapter 6, we really need to go beyond connectivity and think in three-dimensional terms, because real molecules and receptors (as opposed to drawings of them) are three-dimensional objects.

When we move to include the third dimension, we find that these psychoactive molecules fall into three categories:

1. Molecules in which the –C–C–N– side chain is flexible, and thus may adopt any conformation (DMT, psilocybin, serotonin, mescaline)

2. Molecules in which the side chain is also connected to the 2 position of a indole ring and thus forms a third, fairly rigid ring (the β-carboline alkaloids harmine, harmaline, and tetrahydroharmine)
3. Molecules in which the side chain is incorporated into a more complex, rigid ring structure which is connected to the indole 4-position (LSD)

Because the side chain in molecules of the first group is flexible, it can adopt many conformations (shapes), including the shapes of the second and third groups. They are probably capable of binding to the same receptors as the second and third groups, so their three-dimensional shape doesn't give us much help (though their connectivity, a two-dimensional concept, was still a useful clue). Consequently, when thinking in terms of three-dimensional shape, there are really only two unique groups of molecules, the latter two groups.

In these two groups, the indole ring and –C–C–N– chain are important for psychoactivity, but their relative locations in LSD and the β-carbolines are rather different. Recall that for a molecule to bind to a receptor, the various functional groups have to be oriented so that they can interact with complementary functional groups on the receptor (Chapter 6). Because of their different shapes, one would reasonably guess that these two groups of molecules bind to different receptors, or to the same receptor with different strengths (perhaps because of different orientations, or they may bind at entirely different locations on the same receptor). It's also important to remember that LSD has two chiral centers that affect its shape. Figure 7.7 emphasizes the differences in shape between LSD and harmine. Each molecule is shown separately at the left but with similar orientation. On the right is a view of what one gets by overlaying and aligning the indole rings of each molecule. As you can see, the –C–C–N– chain of each molecule points in a different direction. By looking at similarities in connectivity and thinking about the molecule's three-dimensional shape, we have developed some pretty specific hypotheses about the receptor binding process. However, this is about as far as we can go working from the chemical structures and their shapes. We need to go at the problem from the other direction and turn to the serotonin receptors to which these molecules bind.

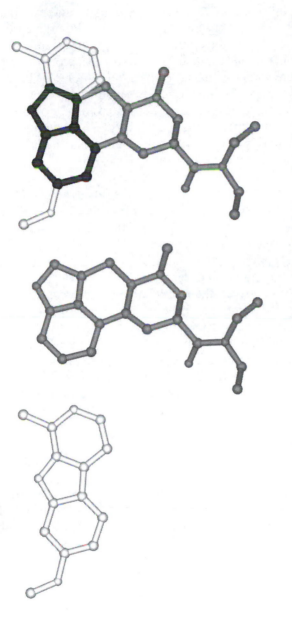

FIGURE 7.7. Comparison of harmine with LSD. Left: Harmine; middle: LSD; right: overlay of the two molecules. In the overlay, harmine is white and LSD gray. The nine black atoms are common to both molecules and were aligned to overlay the two molecules. See corresponding figure in the color plate section.

The research on serotonin receptors is extensive and new material appears regularly. Laboratory investigations of hallucinogenic activity employ several different techniques. In some cases, direct studies investigate how individual molecules bind to a receptor. This method can tell you where and how strongly a particular molecule binds. Another technique is to determine the action that occurs when the molecule binds to a receptor. Does it turn the receptor on or off? This can also be done in a quantitative way. Both of these techniques can be done on either native (naturally occurring) receptors, taken from specific tissues of specific animals, or on cloned receptors created with genetic engineering techniques. Yet another way to investigate hallucinogenic activity is more indirect: one trains rats to respond to a particular molecule, then one substitutes a different molecule to see if it produces the same response. When two drugs give the same behavioral effect, it is assumed that they are acting at the same receptor. This technique is called stimulus control.

I mention these methods in order to point out how hard it can be to make comparisons between the results of different researchers. Different laboratory techniques, sources of receptors, and different animal tissues muddle an already complicated system. Finding human subjects who are willing to take these molecules and then quantifying the hallucinogenic activity is difficult (and for many years such research was not allowed by the government due to the social and political issues surrounding hallucinogenic drug abuse). We cannot be sure that a rat trained to respond to LSD is really experiencing the rat equivalent of human hallucinations. Nevertheless, over time some clear trends have emerged.

At this time there appear to be five or six different types of receptors for serotonin and one serotonin transporter/pump system. Many of the receptor types are actually families of related receptors, so more than ten subtypes may be known, in total. Investigations of hallucinogenic molecules all point to the type 2 receptor family as being most important in producing hallucinogenic effects, with a lesser role played by the 1A receptor. Within the type 2 family, activating the so-called 2A receptor appears to be mandatory for hallucinations. However, a number of studies indicate that the 2C receptor plays some sort of role too.[5]

What happens when we compare the hypothesis previously developed about the common core structures to what is actually known about receptor binding? It has only been in the past couple of years that experiments which can answer this question have been reported in the literature. More work is needed, but the preliminary answer is that the β-carbolines bind to the serotonin 2A receptors in a different manner than LSD, DMT, or synthetic relatives of mescaline (these last three molecules appear to bind similarly to the receptor). This is the same conclusion we reached using basic reasoning about molecular connectivity and shapes, via the overlay diagram in Figure 7.7, as simple as it was.[6] So it would appear that the β-carbolines orient themselves in the receptor binding pocket somewhat differently than the other molecules. While the details of binding for any of these molecules are not known, a different and presumably weaker binding of the β-carbolines would be consistent with the lesser hallucinogenic activity of these molecules.

Understanding the details of these receptors and how molecules bind to them is an important step in understanding how these molecules produce hallucinations. Unfortunately, even if we know exactly how many receptor types there are, where in the brain they are located, what molecules bind to them, and how strongly, we still won't know how hallucinations are produced (although we might be able to enhance them!). The problem is one of connecting molecular events to psychological experiences: We don't really know how groups of neurons work together to form "normal" thoughts or images, so it is presently impossible to explain how such conceptions of reality can be modified to give hallucinations by activating or deactivating certain receptors. This problem is often described with a musical analogy: individual receptors are like a single note on a piano. One needs to hear an entire score in order to enjoy the finished music.

According to M. J. Harner. "We of a literate civilization may get both our religion and our religious proofs from books; persons in non-literate societies often rely upon direct confrontation with the supernatural for evidence of religious reality."[7]

In just the past few years, however, progress has been made in understanding certain spiritual practices that might shed some light on what is happening during a hallucination. Recently devised brain imaging methods that can reveal when various parts of the brain are activated[8] have been used to study people experienced with deep prayer and meditation. People in such states report feelings of tranquility, awe, and ecstasy, as well as having a feeling of oneness with others and the natural world. Combined with data from other studies, a picture is emerging about what happens when people attain these kinds of spiritual states. It appears that portions of the brain whose role is to differentiate "self" from "other" are turned off or isolated from other parts of the brain. This appears to produce the feeling of oneness with nature as the notion of the self dissolves. Although it is still too early to correlate these areas of brain inactivity with changes in the activity of particular serotonin receptors, a very appealing argument can be made that hallucinations induced by ayahuasca have something in common with meditative states. Thus, spirit journeying by an Amazonian shaman may ultimately prove to be a small variation of the neuropsychological event experienced by a Catholic priest deep in prayer, a Buddhist meditating, or a person at a rave, even though the set and setting (to use Leary's terms) vary widely. Some day the molecular events and a more comprehensive understanding of global changes in brain activity may be united to explain it all, but that day appears to be decades off. Although some of these new ideas provide a reasonably satisfying explanation for the experiences of an individual, they don't as yet explain claims of communication between individuals while in these states.[9]

So that is the story of how two plants and their chemicals give rise to spirit journeying, at least as far as the story has been written and can be understood. I hope that you are not too disappointed that a complete answer is not yet available but rather that you are looking forward to hearing about it when it's all figured out. Clearly, there is plenty of work to keep scientists busy for a long time.

GINKGO AND BRAIN HEALTH

The ginkgo tree *(Ginkgo biloba)* has one of the most interesting histories of any plant. It is the only surviving member of a large group, and fossils of ginkgo leaves have been found that are 200 million years old. It is said that at one time the species was nearly extinct but was rescued from Buddhist monasteries in China, where the tree is revered. The use of ginkgo in Chinese herbal medicine[10] goes back nearly 5,000 years, but its benefits have been appreciated only for about the past 40 years in Europe, and perhaps the past 15 years in the United States. Ginkgo is easily one of the most investigated medicinal plants.

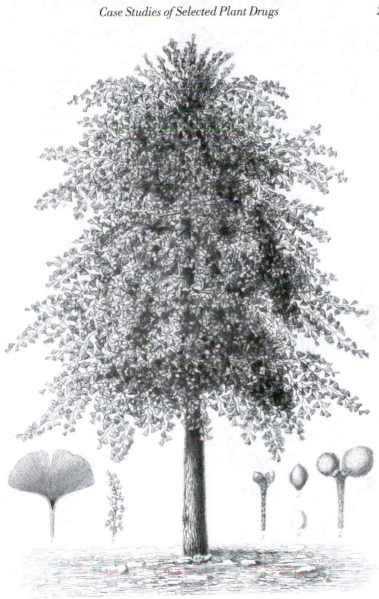

Ginkgo biloba. (*Source: Le Regne Vegetal* divise en traite de botanique, flore medicale, usuelle et industrielle, horticulture theorique et pratique, plantes agricoles et forestieres, histoire biographique et bibliographique de la botanique. Paris: L. Guerin, 1870. Vol. 16, Atlas Iconographique, pl. no. 41.)

The broad medical benefits of ginkgo are related to improved circulation of blood in the small capillaries of the brain, and thus the conditions recommended for treatment with ginkgo are those in which these capillaries are damaged or not working at their optimum. Typically, ginkgo is used to treat conditions related to aging, such as short-term memory loss, inability to concentrate, mood swings associated with anxiety, vertigo, and ringing in the ear (when caused by poor circulation). These clinical symptoms, generally ascribed to "cerebral insufficiency," are associated with decreased blood flow in the small capillaries of the brain, which in turn results in poor oxygen supply to the brain cells. Ample evidence suggests that the effects of ginkgo are protective. A number of studies have investigated whether ginkgo is effective in treatment of the dementia and cognitive problems associated with Alzheimer's disease, and the results are quite encouraging. Other uses for ginkgo have been suggested as well, all related to blood flow problems.[11] Ginkgo has virtually no side effects, but because it improves blood flow, many surgeons require patients to discontinue consumption well before any scheduled surgeries. On the other hand, some studies have shown that ginkgo reduces the inflammation and tissue damage that result from surgery.

The Chemistry and Biology of Ginkgo

Along with its interesting history, the ginkgo tree has some interesting biology. The male and female reproductive organs occur on different trees, so there are male trees and female trees (most tree species have both sexes on the same tree). Although the tree is very beautiful, the female tree produces very odorous berries that make it undesirable for landscaping use in areas where there is foot traffic. Like any plant, ginkgo is a virtual chemical soup of compounds. The medicinally important extract is made from the dried leaves under carefully controlled conditions.[12] The chemical components identified as being responsible for the medicinal effects fall into two categories: flavonoids and terpenes. Based upon extensive research, it is generally agreed that the extract should be concentrated and standardized so that it contains about 25 percent flavonoid glycosides and about 6 percent terpenes. Figure 7.8 shows representative structures of the most important molecules.

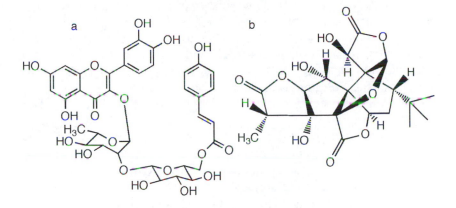

FIGURE 7.8. Bioactive molecules of *Ginkgo biloba*. a: a flavonoid glycoside; b: ginkgolide B.

How Ginkgo Protects the Brain

The neuroprotective activity of ginkgo can be traced to at least three different modes of action. These different modes appear to work in a sort of synergy in that they reinforce one another, adding to the neuroprotective effect.

AntioxidantBehavior

One of these effects is the antioxidant behavior of the flavonoid glycosides, which serve to quench any reactive oxygen species (ROS) present. In Chapter 5 we learned how ROS can damage lipids, DNA, and proteins. As these damaged molecules accumulate, they are re-sponsible for much of what we consider the unfortunate biological aspects of aging. ROS are always present, but the exact amount is a balance between the natural processes that create them, lifestyle choices (diet, smoking), and the efficiency of repair mechanisms. Consumption of ginkgo extract should contribute to one's general health much as any diet high in antioxidant-rich vegetables would. This effect is not unique to the brain, but the brain certainly benefits. The antioxidants in ginkgo, however, have been shown to be espe-cially effective at relaxing the capillaries of the brain, and therefore allowing more blood to flow, which presumably helps one to think better! At least part of this effect is due to the antioxidants interacting with nitrous oxide (NO), a naturally occurring ROS that acts as a hormone or signal molecule to control blood vessels.

In addition to contributing to good general brain health, the flavonoid glycosides of ginkgo can also play a role in more serious acute events such as strokes, including strokes so small that they cannot be clinically detected.[13]

The scenario might go like this: A small capillary or even just a few cells rupture, causing a tiny amount of bleeding in the brain. When cells rupture, they release their contents into the bloodstream. Some of the molecules released act as signals to attract various cells of the immune system, including platelets, a component of the blood which helps clot the blood. As these signals go out, phagocytes and related cells arrive to clean up the mess, and the process of clotting begins. However, as discussed in detail in Chapter 5, phagocytes produce ROS to destroy damaged (or foreign) cells and molecules. The production of ROS can become excessive, particularly as the blood flow slows down due to clotting and the concentration of ROS goes up in the immediate area. This reduced blood flow is known as ischemia, and if it remains relatively minor, it is like an undetected stroke. As a clot increases in size, the result is similar to a chain reaction on a highway following a small accident, with healthy blood cells (cars not involved in the accident) backing up and being caught in the matrix of dead and dying cells (cars involved in the accident). What's happening here is inflammation, with the initial damage creating signals that call in more cells, which in turn create more damage. The cycle is much like that described in Chapter 5 for atherosclerosis, but it has even more in common with the events leading to asthma. Both asthma and ischemia are short-term inflammatory events, whereas atherosclerosis occurs over a much longer period of time before crisis occurs (a heart attack).[14]

The only way out of this situation is to provide a means for stopping the inflammation. Our natural defenses and diet are part of the strategy, but the flavonoid glycosides of ginkgo (see Figure 7.8) are especially potent quenchers of ROS. The diagram in Figure 5.28 shows how they can function in a cycle to repeatedly quench or destroy a wide range of ROS. Many studies have shown that ginkgo flavonoids significantly decrease the amount of damage that occurs in stroke-like situations. Thus, regular consumption of ginkgo extract during one's senior years not only contributes generally to good cerebral blood flow but also provides a reservoir of antioxidants that decreases both the likelihood and severity of strokes.

PlateletActivatingFactor

The second manner by which ginkgo improves circulation in the brain is intertwined with the more general antioxidant effect just described. It involves an important signaling molecule called platelet activating factor, or PAF. PAF is activated in a variety of cells when an inflammatory event occurs, so PAF is involved in the scenario just described, but separately from the production of ROS.[15] However, the two are indirectly linked by their chemistry. Figure 7.9 shows the structure of PAF, which has much in common with the structure of lipids found in membranes, such as those shown in Figure 4.5, especially phosphatidylcholine. However, with its shortened chain, PAF resembles a damaged lipid even more. Compare the structure and general shape of PAF with the damaged lipids illustrated in Figure 5.23. It turns out that many damaged lipids created by the action of ROS can mimic the activity of PAF, which we are about to describe because their shape and structure are so similar.

PAF acts only over short distances because when it is activated, it is brought from the interior of the cells lining the blood vessels to the surface of the cell membrane, where it exerts a variety of effects. The

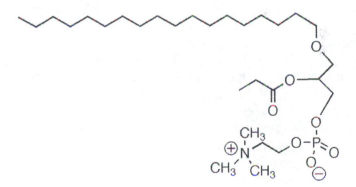

FIGURE 7.9. The structure of PAF. Note the similarity to Figure 4.5 and the damaged lipids depicted in Figure 5.23.

most important is that PAF, sitting on the outside surface of the cells lining a capillary, "catches" and binds to a PAF receptor on circulating platelets. When the PAF receptor binds to PAF (its ligand), other molecules are activated in the platelet that literally cause the platelet to stick to the endothelial cell. This is one of the primary events in the blood-clotting process, and if it can be interrupted, the cascade of events leading to complete blockage (stroke), as well as ROS production, can be diminished (keep in mind that there is a time and a place for blood clotting—we don't want to inhibit the process too strongly!). It turns out that ginkgolide B, shown in Figure 7.8, is a powerful antagonist toward the PAF receptor. An antagonist is a molecule that binds to a receptor and shuts down the normal action of that receptor.[16] In this case, the normal action of PAF is to cause cells to begin sticking together, so an antagonist is a good thing.

Ginkgolide B acts as an antagonist by binding to the PAF receptor at the location where PAF is supposed to bind. Although ginkgolide B can occupy the binding site, it apparently lacks some property that PAF possesses because ginkgolide B fails to turn the PAF receptor on and therefore does not cause cells to stick together. To understand how this can happen, we have to consider both the shape of the ligands (PAF and ginkgolide B) and the details of the receptor. In other words, we have to apply the principles learned in Chapter 6.

On first glance, PAF and ginkgolide B look very little alike (compare Figures 7.8 and 7.9). In addition, because of all the interlocking rings, the two-dimensional picture of ginkgolide B hides its true shape. The left structure in Figure 7.10 is a three-dimensional view of ginkgolide B, which reveals how the rings of the molecule curl back on themselves to create a very compact structure. In contrast to the rather rigid ginkgolide B, PAF, with its long chains of singly bonded atoms, is very flexible (the flexibility issue was discussed in detail in Chapter 3). The bottom line is that PAF can adopt many different conformations or shapes.

Detailed data about the PAF binding site on the receptor are very limited, so it is difficult to map out which functional groups on PAF interact with functional groups on the receptor during the binding process. What we *can* deduce about the receptor comes from studying the relative activity of such molecules as ginkgolide B, its close relatives, and many synthetic derivatives of PAF that have been pre-

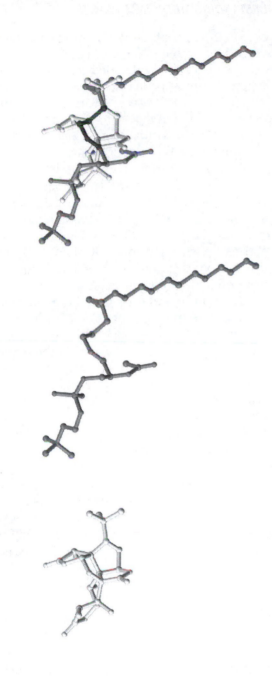

FIGURE 7.10. Comparison of ginkgolide B with PAF. Left: Ginkgolide B; middle: PAF; right: overlay of the two molecules. In the overlay, ginkgolide B is white and PAF gray. The four black atoms are common to both molecules and were aligned to overlay the two molecules. See corresponding figure in the color plate section.

pared.[17] These studies give us clues about the binding process even without the details of functional group interactions.

In this particular case, we have fairly detailed information about several "keys" but not much information about the "lock" (to draw on Fischer's metaphor). We know that PAF is very flexible, that ginkgolide B is rather compact and rigid, and that both bind to the receptor remarkably well. If we use all of the available information and try to match specific atoms of ginkgolide B with particular atoms on PAF, we find that, in spite of their rather different characteristics, a fairly good match can be achieved. By aligning the ring ether oxygen in ginkgolide B with the ether oxygen of PAF, and aligning the nonpolar $(CH_3)_3C-$ group of ginkgolide B with the long nonpolar hydrocarbon tail of PAF, we find that the polar phosphorous group and positively charged nitrogen of PAF are positioned in a rather polar region of ginkgolide B. Thus a very good correspondence in shape and a reasonable correspondence in functional groups can be made between these two keys. We would naturally prefer to have more information about the lock, but such information is not yet available. Figure 7.10 shows the three-dimensional structure of ginkgolide B at left, and the middle structure is a particular conformation of PAF in three dimensions. The good correspondence between these two structures can be seen when they are overlayed or docked, as in the right-hand structure. We know from other data (not given here) that the long hydrocarbon tail is apparently immersed in a membrane, which explains how the $(CH_3)_3C-$ group can be accommodated, since the membrane and hydrocarbon groups are all nonpolar. We also know that the $-OC(=O)CH_3$ group of PAF cannot be much longer or binding will be severely inhibited. Therefore, we can conclude that this group fits into a small binding pocket which limits the size of this chain. This model serves to explain how ginkgolide B can substitute for PAF at the receptor. By occupying the site but not turning the receptor on, ginkgolide B can interrupt the inflammatory cycle described earlier.

GeneRegulation

The third means by which ginkgo may protect the brain has only recently been discovered and is not fully understood. In all organisms the genetic information in DNA is transcribed into messenger RNA (mRNA). In turn, the information coded in the mRNA is translated into proteins, which then serve a variety of functions (see Chapter 4). The information in DNA is located in chunks known as genes, each of which codes for a particular protein with a particular function. However, only certain genes are turned on at any given time in an organism's life, or they are only on in certain tissues.[18] This is a result of regulation; when a gene is turned on we say it is being expressed. The overall scheme is shown in Figure 7.11.

Recent advances in biotechnology permit the monitoring of the expression of many genes at once. It has been discovered that consumption of ginkgo extract by mice increases the expression of certain genes in particular parts of the mouse brain. Genes responsible for proteins with important brain functions, such as transmembrane proteins which handle signaling, and ion channels, which regulate neurotransmission, are expressed at more than three times the normal level when ginkgo extract is consumed. A protein that affects the transport of a hormone, which in turn affects the growth of neurons and plays a role in Alzheimer's disease processes, is greatly increased as a result of ginkgo consumption. Another protein, an enzyme also associated with Alzheimer's, is strongly up-regulated. The parts of the brain studied were the hippocampus, which is the center for learning and memory, and the cerebral cortex, which serves to control speech, memory, and a variety of other functions. Taken together, it is clear that ginkgo extract has a dramatic effect on the levels of important brain proteins by increasing their expression. This recent discovery has really only opened the door to a more detailed analysis of how all of these parts are working together, but it is easy to see that molecules in the ginkgo extract are orchestrating a much more global effect on the brain than had been previously recognized. The alteration of gene ex-

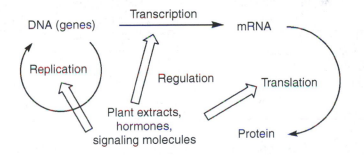

FIGURE 7.11. The flow of genetic information and its potential control.

pression in a particular type of tissue is a great example of an underappreciated effect of medicinal plants. We are likely to see many more examples of this kind of study in the future.[19]

CANCER TREATMENTS FROM PLANTS: INTERRUPTING THE CELL CYCLE

Cancer is certainly one of the most pressing health concerns of people today, especially as people are living longer, and treatments for diseases that used to kill us earlier, such as heart disease, are improving. The term *cancer* is of course very broad, and although all cancers have many things in common, each kind of cancer also has unique characteristics. Some of these characteristics involve the biology of particular cell types, and some involve more practical matters of clinical treatment. It's clear that there will not be *a* cure for cancer but rather *many* cures. Of course, at this point in human history we are really talking about *treatments* for cancer rather than *cures,* in most cases. Drug molecules isolated from plants have been very important in the treatment of cancer. In this section we discuss some of the biology and chemistry of cell division and then see how molecules from plants can be used to alter the natural growth cycle of cells.

The Cell Cycle

One thing that all cancers have in common is that they arise from cells which are growing out of control. In adults, relatively few kinds of cells are actually dividing or growing; those that are growing are cells which need regular replacement. For instance, skin cells and the lining of the intestinal tract (which is technically a skin surface) are constantly being shed and replaced. Hair cells, an extension of the skin, are always growing as well. Because the cellular components of blood are continually replaced, bone marrow, the source of these cells, also grows throughout life. Most other types of cells do not continue to divide once a person reaches maturity. Because cancer represents cells growing out of control, many of the strategies to treat cancer attempt to interrupt the growth cycle of cells. Figure 7.12 diagrams the life cycle of a cell.

Other than the cell types just mentioned, cells spend the majority of their lives carrying out their normal functions.[20] Because they are

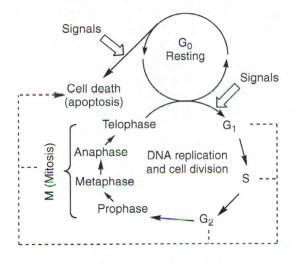

FIGURE 7.12. The cell cycle. See text for explanation.

not dividing, this is termed the *resting phase* (G_0). When (and if) the appropriate signals are received, the cell begins the process of dividing into two cells by synthesizing extra enzymes and building blocks for nucleic acids and proteins (G_1). Next, the cell's DNA is copied (replicated[21]) during the S phase (for synthesis) and additional necessary molecules are readied (G_2). Finally, the cell undergoes mitosis or cell division (M), the process in which the two copies of DNA are pulled to opposite ends of the cell (under the guidance of microtubules, discussed next), and the cell is actually split into two new cells.

With proper staining, the various stages of mitosis can be seen as distinct events under the microscope (known as prophase, metaphase, anaphase, and telophase). After dividing, the cell returns to the resting phase. At some point a cell may receive a signal to die a natural death, a process called apoptosis (the cycle can be redirected by drugs at many points to apoptosis; this is indicated in the figure with a dotted line).[22]

A cell becomes a cancer cell when it receives, internally or externally, the signal to divide too frequently. One strategy in treating cancer has been to address the molecular events that make up this signal so that it can be turned off. Another treatment strategy is to trick the cell into dying prematurely, again by targeting the appropriate signals. These signaling events are of great interest, but they are poorly understood. While there is great potential for cancer treatments in controlling these signaling processes, to date no practical treatments have been developed (at least none that we know of appear to work on the signals). On the other hand, the process of mitosis is relatively well understood, and several plant molecules are known to interrupt the various processes of mitosis. The organization and pulling of the DNA copies to opposite ends of a cell during mitosis is handled by fascinating structures called microtubules, which turn out to be a good target for intervention.

Microtubules

Microtubules are literally tiny tubes that are assembled from just two kinds of protein building blocks. Although they are "micro" in the sense they fit into a cell, they are among the largest assemblies found in cells. The small protein building blocks are called α- and β-tubulin. These two very similar proteins associate with each other to form a complex called a dimer. These dimers in turn form long strings called protofilaments by associating *end to end*. Between 9 and 16 of these protofilaments can associate along their long *edges* to form the microtubule. The construction hierarchy is illustrated in Figure 7.13. The "glue" that holds the microtubule together is the intermolecular forces discussed in Chapter 6 (electrostatic attractions, hydrogen bonding, and hydrophobic forces). A variety of evidence indicates that the α- and β-tubulin are held together rather strongly in the dimer. The forces holding the protofilaments together along their long edges to form the microtubule are somewhat weaker. This is important, because the microtubule must be able to disassemble and reassemble at various stages of cell division, including when the microtubules are pulling the two copies of DNA to opposite ends of the cell, the most important phase. This situation is referred to as "dynamic instability." If the forces holding it together were very strong, the structure would be too stable and would essentially be permanent. In fact, most of the time microtubules are present only during cell division. The rest of the time the components (α- and β-tubulin) are dispersed throughout the cell awaiting the signal to assemble.[23] In some cells, microtubules also play a role in cell movement and mobility. By as-

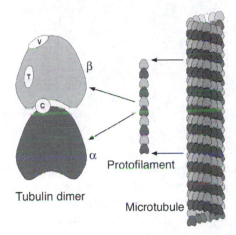

FIGURE 7.13. The structure of microtubules. See text for details.

sembling and disassembling in a synchronized manner, the micro-tubules can impart movement to a cell or to the cilia, small append-ages on the cell which act as propellers.

Plant Drugs That Act on Microtubules

Several molecules isolated from plants have been found to act upon the tubulin dimer and therefore interrupt any further formation of microtubules. By doing so, they stop cell division or mobility and thus have become useful medicines.

Colchicine

Colchicine, Figure 7.14, is an alkaloid isolated from the seeds of the autumn crocus, *Colchicum autumnale,* a plant found in swampy areas in Eastern Europe. The plant is very toxic and can kill if enough is ingested. Colchicine affects microtubule assembly by binding at the junction of the α and β subunits of the tubulin dimer. (The binding site is shown with a C in Figure 7.13. Figure 7.13 is of course merely an illustration that gives a general idea of where the binding site is lo-cated. Much greater detail is known but not needed for our discus-

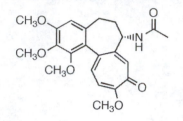

FIGURE 7.14. Colchicine.

sion.) Although the binding site for colchicine involves both subunits of tubulin, it is still possible to form the dimer when colchicine is present. However, the limited evidence available suggests that colchicine wedges itself between the α and β subunits and subtly changes the overall shape of the tubulin dimer, and that this shape change prevents the tubulin dimers from assembling into protofilaments.

Unfortunately, colchicine is too toxic to be used as an anticancer treatment. It has, however, found use since ancient times as a treatment for gout, a very painful condition in which uric acid crystals are deposited in the joints of the foot.[24] Such crystals induce inflammation, which attracts cells of the immune system, which in turn cause more inflammation (recall our discussion of ROS and inflammation in Chapter 5). Rather than affecting cell division, colchicine appears to act by decreasing the mobility of these immune cells. It does this via the tubulin system because, as mentioned, microtubules are also responsible for cell movement.

Paclitaxl

Paclitaxel (Taxol) is a diterpene from the Pacific yew tree (Taxus brevifolia) that has found much use in the treatment of cancer (see Figure 4.36 for the structure). Clinically, paclitaxel has proven particularly useful in breast, lung, testicular, and ovarian cancers. Like colchicine, it acts upon microtubules, but in the case of paclitaxel the effect is to stabilize the completed microtubule and prevent its disassembly, which "arrests" the cell in middivision and leads to cell death. The binding site of paclitaxel on the β subunit is shown in Figure 7.13 with a T. More detailed data show that paclitaxel binds to tubulin at a location which ultimately puts it on the inside (toward the

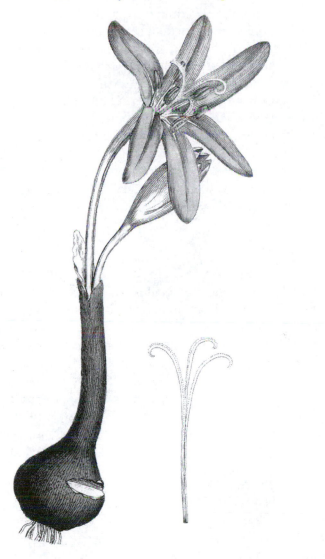

Colchicum autumnale. (*Source:* Woodville, William. *Medical Botany* containing systematic and general descriptions, with pl.s of all the medicinal plants, indige-nous and exotic, comprehended in the catalogues of the material medica; as published by the Royal College of Physicians of London and Edinburgh; accom-panied with a circumstantial detail of their medicinal effects, and of the diseases in which they have been most successfully employed. London: printed and sold for the author by J. Phillips, 1793, Vol. 3, pl. no. 177.)

hollow interior) of the microtubule, and that it acts by strengthening the attractions between adjacent protofilaments. Rather than participating directly in these attractions, however, it appears paclitaxel causes a change in the shape of the β subunit in a way that makes it possible for other parts of the subunit to more effectively interact with adjacent protofilaments. The actions of both colchicine and paclitaxel to alter the shape of the microtubule building blocks are based on the intermolecular attractions discussed in Chapter 6, which in turn affect the shape of the molecules on a large scale. You'll recall that the shapes of much smaller molecules were discussed in Chapter 3. Although the size of the molecules is very different, the same principles are in action in both large and small molecules.

Vinca *Alkaloids*

The final class of plant molecules which we'll discuss that interact with tubulin in some fashion are the *Vinca* alkaloids, a structurally complex group of molecules isolated from various *Vinca* species (Figure 4.12 shows the structure of vincristine). *Vinca roseus* is commonly called the Madagascan periwinkle and is frequently used as a bedding plant because of its attractive flowers. However, few people admiring this plant know its importance in cancer treatment. Vincristine and its close relative vinblastine are used in the treatment of several cancers, especially those of the brain and lung. They have also found application in Hodgkin's disease and non-Hodgkin's lymphoma.

These molecules act by binding to a site on the end of the β-tubulin subunit (marked with a V in Figure 7.13). When this binding site is occupied by a *Vinca* alkaloid, lengthwise growth of a protofilament by the addition of more dimers is prevented. In fact, assembly of microtubules can be prevented by having just one *Vinca* molecule bound at the growing end of an existing protofilament, which means that the amount of drug required is quite low. By stopping growth and recycling of the tubulin dimers, these alkaloids can interrupt the cell growth cycle in the cell division (mitosis) phase and thereby slow the growth of cancer cells.

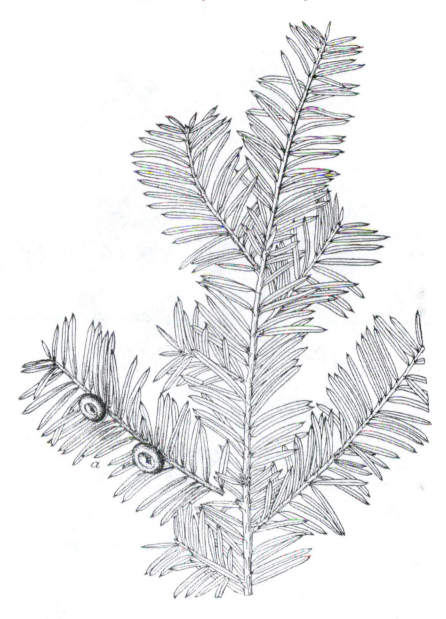

Taxus brevifolia. (*Source:* Sudworth, George B. *Forest Trees of the Pacific Slope.* Washington, DC: U.S. GPO, 1908, p. 195, fig. 76.)

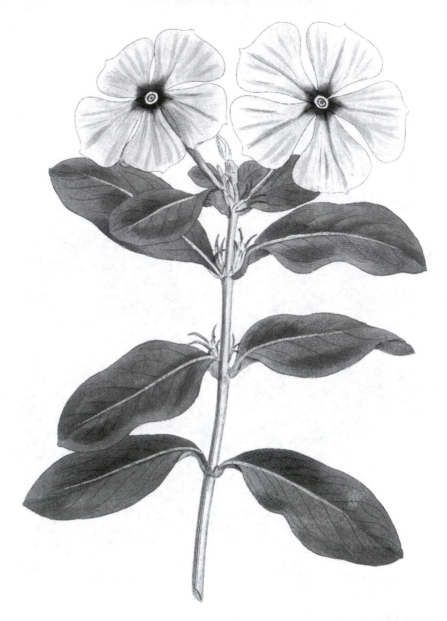

Vinca roseus. (*Source: The Botanical Magazine, or, Flower-Garden Displayed.*
London: printed by S. Couchman for W. Curtis, 1794. Vol. 7, pl. no. 248.)

DNA Replication

Naturally, before the microtubules can direct the copies of DNA into two new cells, those copies must be made. The replication (copying) event is another molecular process that plant molecules can affect to potentially stop the growth of a cancerous cell. Replication is a sufficiently complicated process that it contains many targets for plant drug therapy. We'll begin with a general overview of DNA replication.

You'll remember from Chapter 4 that DNA exists as a double helix—two strands that wind around each other. The amount of DNA in any cell is quite large, and in order to fit within the cell the long sections of double helical DNA are themselves wound into coils. This is referred to as supercoiling. The construction and behavior of common rope provides a good analogy for both the double helix and supercoiling. Most rope is composed of three smaller strands wound around one another. Except for having *three* strands, this is similar to the double helix. Supercoiling can be simulated by taking a length of rope and holding one end in a fixed position. If you then begin twisting the other end in the same direction as the rope is already twisted, you'll find that kinks will eventually form. If you continue twisting, the kinks become tighter and tighter, and the overall length of the rope begins to shorten. This is exactly how DNA is stored in cells. Twists upon twists (supercoiling), while perserving the underlying double helix, allow a very long piece of DNA to fit in a very small cell.

The process of DNA replication begins then with the unwinding of these supercoils to return to "plain old" double helical DNA. Special enzymes called topoisomerases[25] handle this unwinding job (we'll return to them shortly). Next, the double helix itself is unwound by an enzyme called helicase. Once a portion of DNA is totally unwound, enzymes called polymerases[26] begin assembling the new strands of DNA. Eventually, two completely identical (we hope) sets of DNA are created and can be transferred to the two new cells. The process of DNA replication is of course much, much more complicated than the brief description just given. A number of proteins participate, and many events have to occur in a coordinated fashion.[27] However, both topoisomerases and polymerases are interesting targets for plant drugs, because if the work of either can be disrupted, DNA replication is halted and, in turn, mitosis is halted. This is an entirely different way of interupting the cell cycle and stopping cancer than interfering with the assembly of microtubules.

Plant Drugs That Affect DNA Replication

Camptothecin

Camptothecin, which we discussed briefly in Figure 2.7, was isolated from the stem wood of the Chinese tree *Camptotheca acuminata* in 1966. It is the original member of what has become a family of anticancer derivatives which find use in the treatment of advanced colorectal, ovarian, and small-cell lung cancers. The development of this family of drugs faltered early on due to problems with poor water solubility, and then the first water-soluble derivatives that became available proved too toxic for clinical use. Eventually these problems were solved; one of the drugs in current use is irinotecan. Figure 7.15 compares the structure of camptothecin with irinotecan,

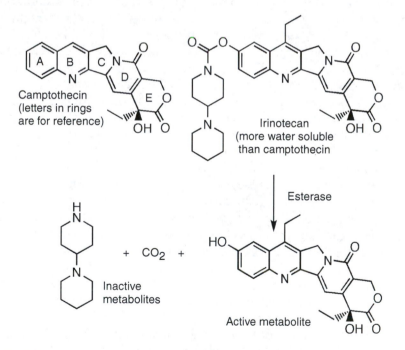

FIGURE 7.15. The metabolism of irinotecan and a comparison to camptothecin.

and shows how researchers were able to use Phase I metabolism to their advantage. Because of the large, polar group on the left end of irinotecan, it is more water soluble than camptothecin, making it practical to give the drug intravenously. However, once administered and in the bloodstream, the esterases of Phase I metabolism (see Chapter 6) cleave off the polar group, giving a metabolite which is 1,000 times more potent than irinotecan.[28]

Once in the bloodstream, and then in a dividing cell, derivatives of camptothecin act by interfering with topoisomerase I (TOP1), one of the DNA supercoiling enzymes just discussed. In its normal function, TOP1 forms a complex with a piece of DNA and helps it unsupercoil (this is usually referred to as "relaxing" the supercoils). It does so by breaking one strand of the DNA, which permits the "tension" in the DNA to be relieved by rotating the broken strand around the intact strand. After unwinding one revolution, TOP1 then rejoins the broken strand of DNA.[29] Camptothecin (and its relatives) interfere with this process by binding to an already formed complex of DNA and TOP1. It stabilizes the complex at the stage where one DNA strand is already cut (camptothecin will not bind to DNA only or to TOP1 only; it must bind to both simultaneously). By itself, this binding is reversible. However, when the enzymes that are busy replicating DNA run into the TOP1/camptothecin/DNA complex, the complex comes apart and the broken strand of DNA is released, leading to apoptosis in S phase; this results in cell death (see Figure 7.12). Interestingly, it has been found that the action of camptothecin is enhanced when DNA bases are nearby that have been damaged by ROS (see Figure 5.25) or when a DNA base pair mismatch is present, which can also result from ROS damage. This observation illustrates how oxidative damage to important biomolecules, as discussed in Chapter 5, has implications for the functioning of the cell. Because ROS-damaged DNA is more susceptible to the action of camptothecin, more DNA strand breaks will occur, which in this case would imply greater anticancer action. This would be a case in which oxidative damage might actually appear be a good thing (and it is—in a test tube). Remember, however, that the evidence indicates ROS damage to biomolecules is a major cause of cancers.

How does camptothecin bind to TOP1 and DNA simultaneously? As in the case of all the other plant drugs discussed in this chapter, scientists have made small changes to the structure of camptothecin and measured the effect on its binding and cell-killing capabilities.[30] These studies determined the structural features that were necessary for activity as well as which parts of the molecule could be modified without losing activity.[31] For instance, all of the rings in camptothecin are necessary for binding to DNA and TOP1, but rings A, B and C (Figure 7.15) can be modified quite a bit, in some cases in ways that improve activity. The cyclic ester of ring E must remain intact, as must the carbonyl group (C=O) in ring D. The chiral center (see Chapter 6) of ring D must have the arrangement shown in Figure 7.15; reversing the positions of the forward and back groups abolishes activity almost completely. These observations serve as clues about the details of how camptothecin binds to its target. They tell us which functional groups are likely to be involved in attractions such as hydrogen-bonding, and give indications about how the overall size and shape affect the fit of camptothecin in the binding site. The information about the chiral center is particularly useful. The alcohol group and the $-CH_2CH_3$ group are not terribly different in terms of size. However, one group is nonpolar, and the other polar and capable of hydrogen bonding. This suggests that the alcohol plays an important part in the binding to DNA and/or TOP1 and therefore must be positioned properly.

These kinds of deductions, although powerful and useful, don't clarify things as much as we would like, because camptothecin is unusual in binding to *tw* molecules at once, a piece of DNA and TOP1. Without additional information, we cannot say what specific role the DNA or the TOP1 plays. Fortunately, an X-ray crystal structure of TOP1 complexed with DNA has been solved, and researchers have modeled how camptothecin would fit into the complex, using some of the key findings just mentioned. Camptothecin binds to the DNA part of the complex by a process called intercalation (see Figure 7.16). Because the GC and AT base pairs of DNA are largely flat, an appropriately sized flat molecule such as camptothecin can slip in between adjacent base pairs and interact with the base pairs above and below it via London forces. (See Figure 4.9 where the base pairs are viewed edge on. The gap between two base pairs, where a flat molecule can slide in, is readily apparent.)[32] After intercalating, the edges of camptothecin stick out from the central part of the DNA helix, and the functional groups on the edges of camptothecin can interact with functional groups from TOP1 or other parts of the DNA. Figure 7.16,

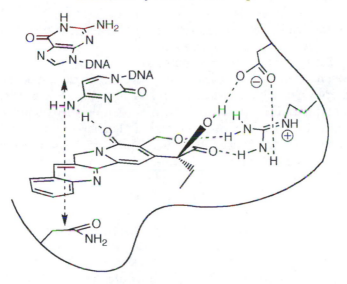

FIGURE 7.16a. Binding of camptothecin to TOP1 and DNA. Structural diagram showing the interactions between the amino acid side chains of TOP1 (shown protruding from the bulk surface of the protein), camptothecin, and portions of the DNA strands. The diagram is expanded along the dotted line for clarity. The dashed lines are hydrogen bonds (see Figure 6.11).

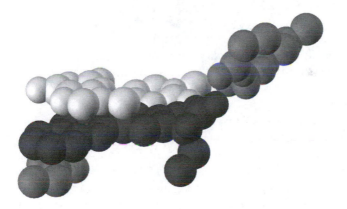

FIGURE 7.16b. Space-filling view of Figure 7.16a. The protein (TOP1) is shown in gray, the DNA strand in white, and camptothecin in black. Note how the flat camptothecin molecule is sandwiched (intercalated) between a group from TOP1 and one of the DNA bases (the other DNA base is at the rear in the same plane as camptothecin). See corresponding figure in the color plate section.

part a, which is expanded in the vertical direction for clarity, allows us to see the details of these functional group interactions. Hydrogen bonding occurs between amino acid side chains from TOP1 and the functional groups in ring E of camptothecin. This explains why the chiral center of camptothecin is so critical to binding. If the alcohol group does not point up (as drawn), a key hydrogen bond is lost, because the $-CH_2CH_3$ group cannot participate in a hydrogen bond. A DNA base hydrogen bonds to the carbonyl group in ring D providing additional stability. This explains why structural variants of campto-thecin that lack the ring D carbonyl group don't bind very well. Finally, a side chain from TOP1 and a DNA base "stack" on the bottom and top, respectively, of the A and B rings of camptothecin (this is the intercalation process). The resulting complex is very stable. Figure 7.16, part b, shows the three-way binding, but this time in space-filling style without expansion, so that the stacking of the groups above and below camptothecin is clearer. Intercalation is a very common and important way in which molecules bind to DNA. We can once again see and appreciate the role of shape, size, and functional groups on binding in this three-way complex.[33]

Other Plant Drugs That Affect Some Aspect of the Cell Cycle

As more and more plants used in traditional folk medicine are studied in detail, scientists are finding that many of them affect the cell cycle. In most cases only hints about their exact mechanism of action are known (whether they affect tubulin, topoisomerases, or something else). A few are mentioned here to give a feel for recent discoveries.

The South American plant commonly known as sangre de grado (blood of the dragon;[34] *Croton palanostigma*) has been used as long as people can remember for wound healing and as a treatment for diarrhea, ulcers, and intestinal inflammation. A recent study has shown that sangre de grado inhibits the growth of stomach and colon cancer cells. The broad effect appears similar to paclitaxel, but more detailed studies are necessary. Podophyllotoxin, a lignan shown earlier in Figure 4.28, is known to inhibit microtubule assembly by binding at the same site as cholchicine. However, podophyllotoxin is too toxic for clinical use against cancer, and researchers have modified the structure slightly to create two useful molecules called etoposide and teniposide. Curiously, in spite of very similar structures, these two drugs don't affect tubulin as podophyllotoxin does, but instead they treat cancer by inhibiting topoisomerase II. Sometimes a very small structural modification changes the entire mode of action.

Several other plants produce molecules that affect topoisomerases. Palmatine and a number of close structural relatives also bind to TOP1 and induce apoptosis, although the mechanism of binding is different than for camptothecin (see Figure 7.17 for the structures discussed in this section). Cryptolepine and neocryptolepine have been isolated from the African climbing shrub *Crptolepis sanguinolenta,* which is used to treat rheumatism, various infections, and malarial fevers. They have been shown to inhibit topoisomerase II. These three molecules, along with camptothecin and sanguinarine (see Figure 4.14), are very structurally similar because they are all largely flat (see Chapter 3). This would lead one to speculate that they may all bind to DNA via intercalation, but this has not been established, except for camptothecin.

Betulinic acid, which is found in many plants but in especially high concentrations in the white birch, *Betula populifolia,* has been found

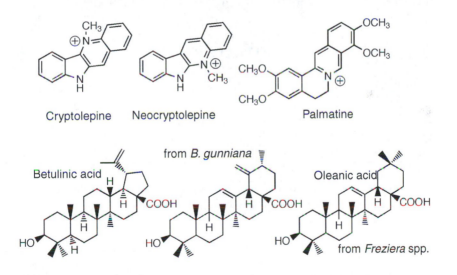

FIGURE 7.17. Molecules that act on various aspects of the cell cycle.

to act on several different types of solid tumors. In at least one case it is known to act by interupting the cell cycle in the G phases. Some derivatives of betulinic acid inhibit the assembly of HIV. Exactly which process and molecule is targeted by these compounds remains to be studied. Finally, compounds isolated from *Baeckea gunniana* and *Freziera* spp. have been found to inhibit an enzyme called DNA polymerase β. This enzyme is responsible for the repair of damaged DNA. Because many anticancer agents (both plant derived and synthetic) damage DNA along the road to stopping cell growth, their effectiveness could be enhanced if DNA polymerase β were inhibited at the same time so that no repair would occur. Thus, administration of a polymerase β inhibitor along with another anticancer agent may prove extremely effective. These last three compounds are all very closely related triterpenoids, as can be seen in the figure. Again, one is tempted to hypothesize that they may all work in a similar manner, but the preliminary evidence is that they have different targets (or perhaps multiple targets). Obviously many interesting discoveries will be made about how plants from traditional folklore work, and much more research must be done to really understand how these molecules work. It is rather ironic that many technologically simple cultures have been using plants with such sophisticated modes of action.

CONCLUSION

In this last chapter, I have attempted to show a few examples of how medicinal compounds found in plants work on a molecular level and dispel the idea that some sort of mystery or magic is taking place. The principles of bonding, the shapes of molecules, intermolecular forces, and other topics from earlier in the book all help us understand the action of these compounds isolated from medicinal plants. How do we go from a shaman in the jungle curing his people with methods that are centuries old to a modern drug or herbal treatment? After reading this book, much of how that journey happens should be clear. I truly enjoy deciphering these wonderous molecular events that stretch to the origins of human culture. I hope that you too have developed a sense of pleasure from our little tour together, and that you now have the knowledge you need to understand medicinal plants.

SUGGESTED READINGS

Ball, P. (2001). *Stories of the invisible: A guided tour of molecules*. Oxford, United Kingdom: Oxford University Press. A very readable general discussion of the molecular world. Although not only about the molecules of life, a great deal of attention is given to them and the processes they mediate. A variety of biochemical processes related to cancer treatment are covered.

Blumenthal, M., Goldberg, A., and Brinkmann, J. (eds.) (2000). *Herbal medicine: Expanded Commission E monographs*. Boston: Integrative Medicine Communications. More detailed information on clinical studies of ginkgo can be found in this book.

DeFeudie, F. V. (1998). Ginkgo biloba *extract (EGb 761): From chemistry to the clinic*. Ullstein Medical Verlagsgesellschaft. This is probably the most comprehensive single work on ginkgo.

Goodman, J. and V. Walsh (2001). *The story of Taxol: Nature and politics in the pursuit of an anti-cancer drug*. Cambridge, United Kingdom: Cambridge University Press.

Harner, M. J. (1973). *Hallucinogens and shamanism*. Oxford, United Kingdom: Oxford University Press, 1973.

Liska, K. (2004). *Drugs and the human body (with implications for society)*, Seventh edition. Upper Saddle River, NJ: Pearson Prentice Hall. A rich resource of information on drugs of recreation or abuse, plus a few other types, placed in a social context. Provides background on drug metabolism, receptors, synapses, and SAR. Quite a bit of technical vocabulary but it is limited chemical detail. Similar in style and approach to Perrine's book but with far fewer chemical structures.

Metzner, R. (1999). *Ayahuasca: Hallucinogens, consciousness, and the spirit of nature*. New York: Thunder's Mouth Press, 1999. A great resource, especially from the experential perspective. Also includes short chapters on the history and science of ayahuasca.

Nencini, P. (2002). The shaman and the rave party: Social pharmacology of Ecstasy. *Substance Abuse and Misuse* 37(8-10): 923-939.

Newberg, A., d'Aquili, E. G., and Rause, V. (2001). *Why God won't go away: Brain science and the biology of belief*. New York: Ballantine. A very readable account of research on the nature of meditative states and the religous and mystical experience.

Perrine, D. M. (1996). *The chemistry of mind-altering drugs: History, pharmacology, and cultural context*. Washington, DC: American Chemical Society. An excellent discussion of the topic; the pharmacology and chemistry is technical here, but the historical and cultural background is extensively researched, complete, and exceptionally readable.

Robbers, J.E. and Tyler, V. E. (1999). *Tyler's herbs of choice: The therapeutic use of phytomedicinals.* Binghamton, NY: The Haworth Herbal Press. More detailed information on clinical studies of ginkgo can be found in this book.

Schultes, R. E. and A. Hofmann (1979). *Plants of the gods: Origins of hallucinogenic use.* New York: Alfred van der Marck Editions.

Shaman's Drum. Many issues of this journal contain articles on ayahuasca (and advertisements for ayahuasca tourism).

Shannon, Benny (2002). *The Antipodes of the Mind: Charting the Phenomenology of the Ayahuasca Experience.* Oxford: Oxford University Press. An excellent discussion of ayahuasca from the firsthand experience of a cognitive psychologist.

Stone, S. and Darlington, G. (2000). *Pills, potions and poisons: How drugs work.* Oxford, United Kingdom: Oxford University Press. A broader treatment of drug action and more technical.

Notes

Chapter 1

1. *Echinacea* is the Latin genus name for the purple coneflower plant. Such Latin plant names are italicized to remind us that they are part of a system of cataloging living organisms. The genus name, but not the species name, is capitalized.

2. I was hoping this word would get your attention. A pharmacognocist works in the field of pharmacognosy. This is one of my favorite words. Its Latin roots involve pharmacy or drugs, and cognition, the act of thinking or knowing. Most people define pharmacognosy as the study of all aspects of naturally occurring medicinal substances.

Chapter 2

1. I first saw this mnemonic in Perrine's *The Chemistry of Mind Altering Drugs*.

2. One of my mentors taught me this, but "lazy" was not meant in a bad way. Rather, the meaning was one of efficiency. Why draw more than necessary? Besides, if we really were lazy and took too many shortcuts, we would have chemical reactions exploding all over the place.

3. The smaller aromatic hydrocarbons do have an odor, which is sometimes pleasant but more often not. The chemist's use of the term *aromatic* is different from the day-to-day common usage of this term. For chemists, it refers to special properties of the benzene ring, not its smell.

Chapter 3

1. However, we define chemical reactions quite broadly. For instance, passing electricity through a material can cause a chemical change.

2. Compounds are made of more than one element, as just stated. The terms *compounds* and *elements* refer to composition. In contrast, the terms *molecules* and *atoms* refer to objects. A molecule may be composed of atoms of different elements or atoms of the same element.

3. Much of physics concerns itself with the behavior of neutrons, protons, and electrons and *their* building blocks. The field of subatomic physics has its own fundamental building blocks, such as quarks and muons, which *are* the smallest building blocks known (for now).

4. Many elements form compounds with oxygen and the halogens like chlorine, so the reaction patterns involving these elements are particularly useful.

5. This simplification is not some sort of cop-out. Only specialists in quantum mechanics theory can deal with it from start to finish. Most professional chemists only need to use the results, as we will.

6. You may have heard of the Heisenberg Uncertainty Principle, which is behind this statement.

7. You can safely use this information to predict the valence electrons of any element except the transition metals, lanthanides, and actinides. A bit more information is needed to deal with these elements, and they are not relevant to our topic.

8. The inert gases are not truly unreactive, but they are extremely reluctant to react. It wasn't until 1962 that someone convinced xenon (Xe) to form a compound with another element.

9. Very often chemists do not draw the lone pairs unless they are needed to make a point. If you check the structures in Chapter 2, you'll see that was the case. This leaves the viewer of a structure to infer the presence of the lone pairs.

10. In some more complex molecules, hydrogen is listed first in the formula, but it is never central because it can form only one bond. In these cases H is usually attached to O. For an example, see the bicarbonate molecule in Figure 3.10.

11. This is a good time to point out that the rules of bonding, which I originally gave you to take on faith, are actually derived from electron configurations and the periodic table. That's one take-home lesson of this section.

12. For reasons we need not consider, carbon cannot make a quadruple bond, only single, double or triple bonds.

13. When a chemist says "proton" you have to listen to the context to determine if he or she means the subatomic particle called the proton, or the ion H^+, which is also called a proton. Using the same name is quite justified because they are the same, but the context is different. A hydrogen atom, with electron configuration $1s^1$ and atomic number 1, has one electron and one proton. If you lose the electron to give H^+, you are left with just a proton.

14. Alternatively, one could extend the common bonding situations I have illustrated to include situations with formal charges. I have done just that and collected the information in Figure 3.12.

15. Another word that chemists use for shape is *geometry.* Sooner or later I will use both terms.

16. Note that for this structure (and for hypericin) I surreptitiously switched back to bond-line notation and stopped drawing in the lone pairs. As discussed in Chapter 2, you'll have to decode the structure and add the lone pairs in your imagination.

17. The study of animals treating themselves with medicinal plants is called zoopharmacognosy.

18. We don't need to worry about the reasons, but one cannot rotate around double or triple bonds.

19. Formulas that can be written in a standard line of text in such a way that the connectivity is clear are called condensed formulas. At some point a molecule gets too complicated to use a condensed formula, and we have to turn to a drawing.

20. We can relate this back to ionic bonding too. You could say that ionic bonds form between elements that have high electronegativity and elements with low electronegativity. This fits perfectly with the idea of electrons being transferred between two elements. The element that wants to gain an electron has high electro-

negativity, and the one that is willing to give up an electron has low electronegativity.

21. This arrow is technically a vector, which has both direction and magnitude properties. This particular vector is called the dipole moment by physicists and chemists; chemists also call it a bond dipole. The word *dipole* implies the separation of two things toward opposite poles. In this case it is charge that is being separated.

22. We can say this without even knowing whether hydrogen is more electronegative than carbon or vice versa. As it turns out, carbon is just slightly more electronegative; this is illustrated in Figure 3.27.

23. I have dodged defining symmetry because its definition can be daunting. Most people have enough of an appreciation for the concept to recognize it when they see it. For example, people generally recognize snowflakes and bow ties as being symmetrical. We also have to be careful that the symmetry of the molecule is not hidden by the particular way a molecule is drawn on paper. Finally, remember that molecules can be flexible, as discussed earlier. Some shapes of a molecule may hide the inherent symmetry and complicate things. These are some of the reasons we are *estimating* polarity.

Chapter 4

1. In fact, the greatest interest in lipids until recently has been to regulate our dietary intake of them in order to avoid such cardiovascular problems as stroke and heart attack.

2. Enzyme names traditionally end in "-ase," making them easy to recognize.

3. Ricin should not be confused with the *oil* expressed from castor beans, which has a long history of use as a laxative and is not toxic. Ricin has been in the news recently as a potential bioterrorism weapon.

4. In the color art section, α-helices are shown in cyan, β-sheets in green, tight turns in blue, and random sections in orange. For further details about these features see the reference section at the end of this chapter.

5. The terpenes are the largest group.

6. Bases are substances that react with acids, which are proton (H^+) sources. The earliest definition of alkaloids did include their behavior as bases; the word *alkaloid* is derived from an Arabic word *alkalai*, which means "base."

7. Basicity is a property that is often included in the definition of the term *alkaloid*. However, sanguinarine is an example of an alkaloid that does not act as a base, because the nitrogen atom in sanguinarine has no lone pair and thus cannot accept a proton.

8. The alkaloids are even more concentrated in the roots. Tyler (*Herbs of Choice*, 1999) recommends against any use of comfrey. Commercial samples are often contaminated with even more toxic species, and alternatives are readily available.

9. Cocaine does have some legitimate medical uses, though they are rare. Snorting a drug is more officially known as insufflation.

10. Protonated and deprotonated forms are possible for most alkaloids. See the discussion under the introduction to the alkaloids in this chapter.

11. Platelet aggregation is part of the blood clotting process, which one really shouldn't inhibit too much! However, it is also part of the process by which undesired clots form in the small vessels of the brain (leading to stroke) or in the narrowed vessels of the heart (leading to a heart attack), so some inhibition can be desirable.

12. Anthocyanidins are the aglycones of anthocyanins. The glycosides of flavonoids do not have a special name.

13. The seeds of the horse chestnut have similar uses, but the active compounds in the seeds appear to be triterpene glycosides.

14. An epimer is a molecule that is different at one of several chiral centers. These concepts are discussed in Chapter 5.

15. Technically they are thioglycosides because the sugar molecule is linked to the aglycone through a sulfur atom.

16. *Hydrolysis* means breaking down (-lysis) by the action of water (hydro-).

17. The glucosinolates, for example, are thioglycosides in which a sulfur atom links the two parts of the molecule.

18. With more gentle isolation procedures and more sophisticated methods of analysis, it has become apparent that many more compounds exist as glycosides than was originally appreciated.

19. And you wouldn't want to confuse any of these compounds with rutin, which is a different flavonoid glycoside.

20. Do not confuse this group with lignins, which are entirely different molecules that help bind cellulose chains together to make wood.

21. Modification starting from a compound found in nature is called semisynthesis and is generally much more efficient than trying to make the compound from scratch.

22. *Echinacea* is the fifth best selling herbal remedy in the United States.

23. Dimers are molecules formed by the linking of two molecules. Sometimes the linkage is via a covalent bond; other times (for instance with proteins) the linkage involves weak intermolecular forces.

24. Hydrolysis is a fairly broad term and should not be taken to mean that merely adding water causes these compounds to break down. Often, acid or base, possibly along with heat, is needed.

25. Ironically, the anthocyanidins are produced by hydrolysis. However, the conditions required for this hydrolysis are slightly more vigorous than those required for the hydrolyzable tannins.

26. Some essential oils that have medicinal properties include lavender, peppermint, sage, bergamot, wormwood, and eucalyptus. You will almost certainly recognize some of these as cooking spices and flavoring agents. For many years it was thought that the role of spices was to cover the odor of spoiled food. We now know that many spices also provide antibacterial and antioxidant properties.

27. Lactone common names often end in *-olide*. Don't confuse this with *-oside,* which refers to glycosides.

28. Other species in the ecosystem would be at peril too, such as the northern spotted owl.

29. Note that diosgenin has only 27 carbon atoms due to the loss of carbons in the final stages of its biosynthesis.

Chapter 5

1. It would also depend upon the amount of the medicinal substance in the leaves, which in turn depends upon time of harvest, genetics, soil quality, any processing such as drying, and so forth.

2. Most molecules dissolve better if the temperature of the solvent is higher. However, high temperatures can also cause some molecules to decompose, so raising the temperature is not always a good idea.

3. Drinking tea will affect the entire body, which would be a systemic rather than local effect.

4. Unfortunately, we don't have space in this book to discuss how one goes about identifying potentially useful plants. For more information, see *Plants, People, and Culture* by Balick and Cox.

5. I have snuck the definitions of acids and bases into this text: Acids donate protons; bases accept them. When a molecule is dissolved in water, the pH of the solution is a measure of its acidity or basicity. The pH scale runs from 0 to 14 with 7 being neutral. Values below 7 indicate an excess of protons and acidic conditions. Values above 7 indicate a deficit of protons and basic conditions. A deficit of protons also corresponds to an excess of hydroxide ions, HO^-.

6. When we discussed polarity it was in terms of partial charges due to electronegativity. A full formal charge has an even more dramatic effect on polarity.

7. It wouldn't really be quite pure, because the coniine is accompanied by several other alkaloids in minor amounts.

8. In reality, spots often overlap. Sometimes changing the mobile phase (solvent) will prevent this, but not always.

9. One downside of bioassay work with plants is that one is likely to "rediscover" some known compounds that have biological activity. Recently, techniques have been developed to quickly "dereplicate" or identify already known compounds so that further time is not wasted in purifying them.

10. Electromagnetic radiation behaves like a wave, and it can be described in terms of its wavelength, frequency, and energy. As frequency goes up, wavelength goes down, and vice versa. The energy of a wave is proportional to its frequency: the higher the frequency, the more energy that wave carries.

11. This is called the functional group region. The area below $1,500$ cm^{-1} is called the fingerprint region because it is generally unique for each molecule. Police agencies can use the fingerprint region of the IR spectrum to identify illicit substances.

12. If you don't have a molecular formula, finding the structure is more difficult and would require methods we will not discuss. However, the logic employed is exactly the same; there are just different clues.

13. If there is an aromatic ring (a phenyl group, perhaps substituted), this by itself produces an IHD of four (three double bonds and a ring). This can be handy to keep in mind. For instance, if you calculate an IHD of five, and propose an aromatic ring for your structure, then you have only one more IHD unit to account for, which could be in the form of a ring or a double bond (but not a triple bond, which requires two IHD units).

14. All carbon atoms have six protons; the number of neutrons varies from six to eight. Atoms with varying numbers of neutrons are called isotopes.

15. Most people associate the word *nuclear* with damaging and polluting radiation. However, as we have seen, *radiation* is a broad term which includes many things that are generally harmless (and some that are not).

16. There is much more to symmetry than what I have stated. In addition, we have to be careful in drawing conclusions, because a symmetric molecule may be *drawn* so that it appears asymmetric. It is very helpful to use a model of the molecule when looking for symmetry.

17. Counting unique environments based upon symmetry is tricky. In most cases you must take into account the three-dimensional shape of the molecule, as well as the possibility of rotation around single bonds, which "averages" the position of atoms for symmetry purposes. Again, a model is exceptionally helpful.

18. A major marketer of herbs advertises that each lot is checked by TLC, although they give it a fancier name.

19. Other terms that have been used for ROS include oxyradicals and toxic oxygen free radicals.

20. Concentration is defined as the amount of a substance in a certain volume.

21. Oxidative burst is probably the better term, though both are used. Oxygen uptake is increased in this event, but the extra oxygen consumption is not used to react with sugar molecules in the process of digestion, which is what respiration usually refers to.

22. NADPH stands for nicotine adenine dinucleotide phosphate; the H on the end actually represents a hydrogen atom.

23. There are other causes of fever as well.

24. We think of digestion in the usual sense as occurring in our stomach and intestines. What occurs there is only part of the process. The real harnessing of the energy in food occurs in all of our cells, but especially in our muscles.

25. Two percent may not seem like a large amount, but more than a billion oxygen molecules are consumed by a cell in a single day. Two percent of that kind of number is a lot of ROS leaking out and causing trouble.

26. I am speaking of radiation such as that found in X rays and nuclear bombs. The changes observed in aging are exactly the changes observed upon exposure to low levels of radiation.

27. The steps of initiation, propagation, and termination are not restricted to lipid molecules. This section is a good place to introduce and emphasize them because the steps are well studied for lipids, but they occur with all ROS reactions.

28. The inside and outside of the cell membrane are different, and lipids do not migrate or flip from the outside to the inside very often. Lateral movement—that is, movement within the two-dimensional outer or inner layer—is normally rapid.

29. Food manufacturers have recently been under pressure to remove "trans fats" from their products, because of their effect on the human cardiovascular system.

30. Cells also gain protection from ROS by compartmentalizing different processes. As mentioned, the electron transport chain and consumption of oxygen occurs in the mitochondrion, which is a separate structure within the cell. If this process were not contained, the damage from ROS would surely be much higher. As it is, the membranes of the mitochondrion take quite a beating from the internally gen-

erated ROS, and mitochondrial damage is another good measure of the aging process.

31. Perhaps double the risk may not seem so bad, but consider how you would feel about monthly bills that were twice normal.

32. Vitamin C is also important in maintaining healthy connective tissue independent of its role as an antioxidant. Its absence leads to scurvy, in which muscles deteriorate.

33. Studies of antioxidant properties by different researchers using different methods are hard to compare. This list includes items that larger studies have identified as good antioxidants. It is not simple to rank foods or individual molecules by a universal standard, and in fact it may be unwise to do so, as some studies demonstrate that mixtures of antioxidants are important.

34. LDL particles are composed of phospholipids, fatty acids, triglycerides, cholesterol, vitamin E, and a protein called apo B. These molecules can be damaged as described earlier, except for the vitamin E, which serves a protective role.

Chapter 6

1. Recall that in Chapter 4 we discussed chemical kinetics, which was the rate or speed of a chemical reaction. Dissection of the word pharmacokinetics gives two concepts: drugs and rate.

2. Medicinal chemists have a rule of thumb that says that if a molecule has more than 5 NHs and OHs combined, or more than 10 Os or Ns combined, the molecule is unlikely to pass through membranes and be a useful drug. You may recognize this rule as a way of stating the shortcuts for estimating polarity, discussed in Chapter 3.

3. The origins of the word *hydrolysis* are *hydro-,* meaning "water," and *-lysis,* meaning "breaking apart." Thus, hydrolysis is a chemical reaction that uses water to break another molecule apart.

4. A simple definition of oxidation is that it involves adding oxygen atoms to a molecule.

5. Isozymes are enzymes with the same function that differ slightly in their amino acid composition and in the efficiency with which they will process various molecules.

6. Monoamine oxidase was named for the reaction of monoamines, which are amines with one carbon group attached to the nitrogen atom. However, later researchers discovered that MAO's action was not restricted to monoamines but was much broader.

7. For example, when you are frightened, your brain causes your adrenal glands to release adrenaline, which in turn affects nearly every cell in your body.

8. Enzymes and receptors are very large protein molecules—far larger than their substrates or ligands.

9. The lock and key analogy was first put forth by the chemist Emil Fischer in 1894. He was also responsible for most of the early discoveries about amino acids, carbohydrates, and nucleosides (the building blocks of RNA and DNA).

10. The hydrogen bond is terribly misnamed. *It is not a bond* and involves only those hydrogen atoms that are bonded to electronegative atoms.

11. Although the discussion of chromatography in Chapter 5 used the general idea of polarity to explain the separation of molecules, the careful reader will realize that the more detailed interactions described here also apply to chromatography.

12. See the section Using Acid-Base Behavior in Extractions in Chapter 5, and Figure 6.4, for more details.

13. The binding site of an enzyme is frequently called the active site.

14. An inhibitor is an enzyme substrate that binds but won't undergo reaction. There is analogous terminology for receptors. The ligand is the normal or natural molecule that binds to the receptor. An agonist is a molecule that increases receptor activity; an antagonist decreases receptor activity.

15. *Chiros* is the Greek word meaning "hand."

16. *Enantiomer* is a term from Greek meaning "opposite."

17. A 50:50 mixture of two enantiomers is called a racemic mixture.

18. The R isomer costs about five times as much as the mixture.

19. When there is more than one chiral center in a molecule, the situation does get more complicated than if there is only one chiral center. However, the general conclusion that chirality matters is a universal principle.

Chapter 7

1. Quite predictably though, recent years have seen a growth in "ayahuasca tourism" in which people travel to Amazonia (or clandestine sites in urban U.S. cities) to experience ayahuasca. Some of these people are no doubt genuinely seeking personal enlightenment or healing, but others are probably merely interested in a drug trip.

2. At times a patient does drink the ayahuasca in an effort to self-help, to train as an *ayahuasquero* independently, or because the shaman requests it. The Amazonian use of ayahuasca is not limited to shamans in a healing context. It is used as part of the apprenticeship to become a shaman and for personal understanding as well. Small group sessions whose purpose is community enlightenment are also common.

3. The word *psychedelic* is derived from the Greek *psyche,* meaning "mind" or "soul," and *dellos,* meaning "revealing" or "revelation."

4. It's less complicated as long as one considers only one receptor at a time. Any real therapy would have to consider multiple receptors interacting to give some sort of net outcome.

5. Involvement of these receptors is based upon a consensus of many studies. For any particular molecule or family of related molecules, other receptors may be involved, including receptors not responding to serotonin. For example, LSD binds to dopamine and epinephrine receptors in addition to several serotonin receptors.

6. Generally, a simpler idea/theory that explains the data is preferred over a more complex one; this is known as Occam's Razor.

7. *Hallucinogens and Shamanism,* Oxford University Press, 1973.

8. These methods include functional magnetic resonance imaging (fMRI) and positron emission tomography (PET).

9. Some anthropologists have offered a hypothesis about shamanism that many will find offensive. It has been suggested that shamanistic mind states are actually an extension of a schizotypal personality disorder, and that early figures in modern reli-

gions may have also been schizotypal. The original suggestion along these lines, since modified somewhat, is due to Julian Silverman (1967) in his article "Shamans and Actue Schizophrenia" in *American Anthropologist* 69: 21-31.

10. When the long use of ginkgo is cited, it is frequently unrecognized that the ancient Chinese used the seeds. The use of the leaves, which are now accepted to be the more potent part, is relatively modern. The seeds contain relatively more toxins; the toxins in the leaves are removed by processing.

11. Ginkgo is one of the top-selling herbs in the world, perhaps because people are living longer and encountering more frequently the conditions that ginkgo treats.

12. It is impractical to use the leaves from the tree directly because the active ingredients are not sufficiently concentrated. For the commercial extract, ginkgo trees are grown in large groves and the leaves harvested mechanically. This is one reason why the use of the leaves is a modern phenomenon.

13. These small undetected strokes may over time cause the damage and cell death that are ultimately responsible for the mental decline seen with aging.

14. Although ischemia is in principle a short-term event, investigations have shown that the period of time after a blockage is cleared and the blood begins to flow again is one of high ROS production. This phase is called reperfusion because oxygen is once again available to the cells that were starved for it, and oxygen is the ultimate source of most ROS.

15. PAF is involved in any inflammatory event such as allergy, or the processes of atherosclerosis. Some of the lipids in damaged LDL particles are structurally very similar to PAF.

16. The opposite of an antagonist is an agonist. Agonists and antagonists sometimes bind to receptors at a special site that is separate from the binding site for the natural ligand. In this case they exert their action by what amounts to a remote control of the main binding site, which changes its shape and thus its ability to accept the normal ligand.

17. It should not surprise you that a great deal of effort has gone into developing drug molecules that stop the action of PAF.

18. For example, certain genes and their proteins might be needed only in a liver cell, so these genes are "off" in brain cells. All cells, however, have the same set of DNA.

19. This kind of gene regulation is an extension of the observation that drugs can induce the enzymes that metabolize them, as was discussed in Chapter 6 for the enzyme CYP. In this case, the drug is up- or down-regulating genes that are unrelated to the metabolism of the drug itself.

20. For example, they could function as muscle, secrete digestive juices, carry a nerve impulse, or transport oxygen.

21. If you compare Figures 7.11 and 7.12, DNA replication is occuring during mitosis. All other events depicted in Figure 7.11 occur primarily during the G_0 (resting) phase, which indicates that the idea of resting is not quite accurate.

22. An unnatural cell death due to damage is called necrosis.

23. The story of microtubules here is rather simplified. Other proteins besides the tubulins are involved in the assembly of the tubules.

24. Ongoing treatment of gout with colchicine requires about 1 mg per day; a single 10 mg dose will cause death in about a week.

25. The name comes from the science of topology, which deals with surfaces. A Mobius strip is a familiar example of a surface related to the supercoiling of DNA.

26. This name translates to "polymer making enzyme." Remember that DNA is a polymer of sugars, bases, and phosphate.

27. For example, the unwound DNA has to be clamped in place, short pieces of DNA glued together, mistakes fixed, and so forth. Each of these events typically involve several proteins and/or enzymes, all of which could be a target for drug therapy.

28. Irinotecan is properly termed a prodrug. It's not really active until is is metabolized.

29. The action of TOP1 is similar to what happens if you take a piece of rope under heavy load and cut just one of the three strands. The rope will partially unwind. The difference is that TOP1 can put DNA back together, but the rope is of course ruined.

30. Remember that these kinds of analyses are called structure-activity relationships (SAR). We considered this method in detail in our discussion of ayahuasca, and while we didn't emphasize it, the same kinds of studies have been performed with ginkgolide B and PAF, and with such molecules as paclitaxel and vincristine. The same concept was also at work in Chapter 6 when we discussed inhibitors of succinate dehydrogenase.

31. For a molecule to become a practical drug, there must be some parts which can be modified to affect solubility, and so forth. If you compare irinotecan with camptothecin in Figure 7.15, you'll see that adding a large polar group at one end of the molecule did not reduce the desired activity but did make the molecule more water soluble.

32. Intercalation is a very common mode for binding a flat molecule to DNA. Many molecules consisting of two to four aromatic rings can bind DNA in this manner.

33. This three-way complex of TOP1, DNA, and camptothecin is not quite the classic intercalation situation, because only one DNA base stacks onto camptothecin, with protein on the other side. The classic situation is to have DNA bases stacked on both surfaces of the drug molecule.

34. So named for its bright red sap which is obtained by making shallow cuts in the bark.

Glossary

Terms set in small capital letters have their own entry in the glossary. Some classes of compounds are discussed in Chapter 4 and are not listed here.

acid: A substance that can donate PROTONS, which are also known as hydrogen IONS (H+).

active site: The portion of an ENZYME where the SUBSTRATE binds.

ADME: Absorption, distribution, metabolism, and excretion (refers to how drugs travel through the body).

adulterant: An undesirable COMPOUND found in a commercial product; a contaminant.

aglycone: The nonsugar portion of a GLYCOSIDE.

agonist: A LIGAND that enhances the response of a RECEPTOR. Compare to ANTAGONIST.

anion: A negatively charged ION.

antagonist: A LIGAND that decreases the response of a RECEPTOR. Compare to AGONIST.

apoptosis: The process of programmed or planned cell death. Compare to NECROSIS.

aqueous: Dissolved in, or pertaining to, water.

aromatic: A term used to describe a MOLECULE with chemical behavior similar to benzene, which is the simplest aromatic COMPOUND. Although most molecules considered aromatic do have an odor, it is generally not pleasant.

atherosclerosis: A cardiovascular disease in which the walls of the blood vessels thicken, eventually impeding proper blood flow.

atom: The smallest unit of an ELEMENT, consisting of a NUCLEUS containing PROTONS and possibly NEUTRONS, which is surrounded by ELECTRONS.

atomic number: The number of PROTONS in the NUCLEUS of an atom. This also determines the identity of the ATOM/ELEMENT.

atomic symbol: A one- or two-letter abbreviation denoting a particular ELEMENT.

base: A substance that can either donate HO⁻ IONS or accept hydrogen (H^+) IONS (also known as PROTONS).

best fit line: A line which best represents the trend of the individual point values in a CALIBRATION CURVE.

bioassay: A method for measuring the response of biological systems (creatures or cell cultures, for example) to chemicals.

blood-brain barrier: The name given to the MEMBRANES which line the brain capillaries and thus isolate the brain from MOLECULES in the bloodstream.

boat: A shape of the cyclohexane MOLECULE resembling a boat; typically the molecule must be forced into this position because it is not as stable as the alternative, called the CHAIR. Can also apply to any SATURATED six-membered ring embedded in a more complex structure.

bond: An attraction between two ATOMS. Can be further classified as IONIC or COVALENT.

bond angle: The angle formed between three ATOMS that are bonded together.

bond dipole: *See* DIPOLE MOMENT.

brand name: An easily remembered name that can be trademarked. Created by drug companies in part to avoid using complex chemical nomenclature.

caged radical: A RADICAL trapped in the area it was created; as a result, it is very unreactive. Compare with FREE RADICAL.

calibration curve: A graph relating the CONCENTRATION of a substance to a response by some kind of instrument. By taking known concentrations, and measuring their responses, a BEST FIT LINE can be created. The response of an unknown can then be correlated with its concentration.

cancer: A disease in which cells grow in an uncontrolled fashion and eventually overwhelm the body with their needs.

carbon-13 nuclear magnetic resonance spectroscopy: A SPECTROSCOPIC technique that can identify the number and types of unique carbon ATOMS in a structure.

catalyst: Something which speeds up the rate of a reaction.

cation: A positively charged ION.

cell culture: A technique in which cells from a specific part of an organism are grown in vitro for experimentation and observation, for instance in a BIOASSAY.

chain reaction: A series of reactions which are, in theory, self-perpetuating, since the products of one reaction are the reactants in the next. *See* PROPAGATION.

chair: A shape of the cyclohexane MOLECULE which resembles a chair. Can also apply to any SATURATED six-membered ring embedded in a larger structure. This shape is preferred over the BOAT.

chemical reaction: A chemical change in which BONDS are broken and/or made so that the ATOMS are present in different CONNECTIVITIES after the reaction.

chemical shift: The location of an NMR peak, reported in parts per million (ppm). Used to determine the types of BONDS and FUNCTIONAL GROUPS present.

chemotactic substance: A MOLECULE released from a cell, often when damaged, that attracts other cells. One way by which cells communicate with each other.

chiral: A term describing an object which has a nonsuperimposable mirror image. From the Greek word for *hand*.

chromatogram: A graph representing the results of a CHROMATOGRAPHY experiment. Generally some kind of instrument response, in the form of peaks, plotted versus time.

chromatography: A collection of techniques by which MOLECULES can be separated from one another. In some forms, the intent is to separate for the purpose of isolating usable amounts. In other forms, the purpose is to separate and quantify.

cis: A term referring to the arrangement of groups on a double BOND in which the major or largest groups on each end of the double bond are on the same side. Compare to *TRANS*.

clinical trial: A BIOASSAY conducted on people to determine if a drug candidate will be effective and practical.

column chromatography: A form of CHROMATOGRAPHY in which mixtures of MOLECULES to be separated are passed through a column (tube) containing silica gel or a similar STATIONARY PHASE with the aid of a SOLVENT (the MOBILE PHASE).

common name: A convenient name used for a chemical, plant, or animal instead of its complex, technical name.

complex: Two MOLECULES that have loosely associated with one another via intermolecular attractions. The process of complexation is nearly synonymous with COORDINATION.

compound: A substance composed of two or more ELEMENTS.

concentration: A measure of the amount of a substance dissolved in a given volume of SOLVENT.

condensed formula: A textual chemical formula written so that the connectivity is clear. Compare with MOLECULAR FORMULA. It is not possible to write a condensed formula for many COMPOUNDS.

conformer/conformation: A type of ISOMERISM due to the rotation around a carbon-carbon single BOND.

connectivity: The order in which ATOMS are bonded together in a MOLECULE.

constitutional isomers: *See* STRUCTURAL ISOMERS.

coordination: The situation where two MOLECULES associate with each other due to intermolecular attractions. Coordination is nearly synonymous with COMPLEXATION.

covalent bond: A BOND created between two ATOMS when they share ELECTRONS in order to fill their VALENCE ORBITALS.

cross-link: A COVALENT BOND between distant parts of a large MOLECULE like a protein, or a covalent bond between an EXOGENOUS MOLECULE and a biomolecule.

diatomic element or molecule: An ELEMENT that exists in nature in the form of two of its ATOMS bound together.

diffusion: The process by which MOLECULES tend to migrate throughout a container (such as a flask, a cell, or an organ) so that the molecules are spread out evenly.

dimer: A MOLECULE composed of two structural units. The units may be held together by COVALENT BONDS or by weak intermolecular forces (as is typical for protein dimers).

dipole moment: A VECTOR that indicates the direction and magnitude of the separation of charge in an individual COVALENT BOND or an entire MOLECULE.

disulfide bridge: A connection between two protein structures or within a single protein through a BOND between the sulfur ATOMS of two different cysteines (one of the amino acids). A type of CROSS-LINK.

DNA: Deoxyribonucleic acid; the genetic material responsible for storing all information needed to create and operate an organism.

double helix: The shape taken on by DNA; consists of two intertwining strands with phosphate backbones and pairs of bases.

duet rule: An unofficial rule! When forming COVALENT BONDS, hydrogen atoms will try to have two ELECTRONS around their NUCLEUS for stability. Compare to the OCTET RULE.

electromagnetic radiation: A term referring to various forms of light, all of which have WAVE properties and behave simultaneously as electrical and magnetic fields. The light we see is but one form.

electron: A negatively charged subatomic particle which exists outside the NUCLEUS. Used to form BONDS with other ATOMS.

electron configuration: The specific arrangement of ELECTRONS in their ORBITALS around the NUCLEUS of an atom; responsible for the specific bonding properties of an ELEMENT.

electron transport chain: A series of proteins located in the inner membrane of a MITOCHONDRION. Responsible for releasing ENERGY from the ELECTRONS in chemical BONDS in a controlled manner during the last stage of cellular respiration.

electronegativity: The property of an atom that determines how strongly it draws the ELECTRONS of a BOND toward itself.

element: A substance that cannot be broken down into a simpler substance while still retaining its fundamental chemical and physical properties.

eluant: The liquid that flows through and drips out of a LIQUID CHROMATOGRAPHY experiment. Generally collected in test tubes in portions called FRACTIONS.

emulsion: A mixture of two substances suspended in one another.

enantiomers: A pair of MOLECULES which are mirror images of each other and are nonsuperimposable.

endogenous: A term describing a MOLECULE that is normally found in the body; a naturally occuring chemical. Literally an "insider." Compare to XENOBIOTIC or EXOGENOUS.

endothelial cell: A cell lining the blood vessels or the inside of other internal organs. Literally means "inside skin."

energy: The ability to do work, due either to an object's motion (kinetic energy) or its position (potential energy). The energy in a chemical BOND is potential energy. The energy carried by a MOLECULE in motion is kinetic energy.

enzymatic defenses: A system of ENZYMES designed to prevent cellular damage by catalyzing the destruction of ROS.

enzyme: A biological CATALYST composed of protein; speeds up the RATE OF REACTION of a SUBSTRATE.

epimer: A MOLECULE whose stereochemistry is different at only one of several CHIRAL centers.

epithelial cell: A skin cell.

equlibrium: A system in which two MOLECULES or COMPLEXES of molecules or CONFORMATIONS of a molecule are found in a particular ratio relative to each other. When the amount of one species is disturbed, the system responds to restore the original ratio. The two species forming the system must be related by a chemical change (a reaction or complexation process) or a change in shape (a conformational process).

essential oil: An oil extracted from a plant, generally with medicinal properties or perfumery potential.

ethnobotany: The study of how cultures use plants for medicinal and material purposes.

exogenous: A term describing something which is not normally found in the body; an "outsider." Compare with ENDOGENOUS.

extraction: The process in which substances of interest are removed from their natural environments. Normally the substances are at least partly concentrated and purified during an extraction.

fat: Another name for a LIPID.

fatty acid: A carboxylic acid with a long, unbranched chain of carbons (usually ten or more and an even number); the building block of many lipids.

fingerprint region: The region in an IR spectrum below $1,500 \text{ cm}^{-1}$ (wavenumbers) which is unique to each molecular structure.

fluid mosaic model: A model describing biological membranes. "Fluid" refers to the semiliquid state of the LIPID bilayer. "Mosaic" reflects the fact that the membrane is composed of a variety of types of LIPID MOLECULES as well as a variety of PROTEINS which float in the bilayer.

foam cell: An enlarged cell created when a MACROPHAGE engulfs damaged LDL particles during ATHEROSCLEROSIS. A mature foam cell contains parts of dead cells, damaged LDL particles, and collagen and calcium deposits.

formal charge: The charge on an atom in a MOLECULE that results from the atom having more or less ELECTRONS around it than it possesses as a free atom.

fraction: One of several tubes of ELUANT collected from a CHROMA-TOGRAPHY experiment. Some fractions may contain only SOLVENT, but others may have compounds of interest dissolved in them.

free radical: A freely mobile RADICAL.

freebasing: The process of treating an alkaloid salt with a basic substance to deprotonate the nitrogen to liberate the "free base." The freebase is often absorbed more readily by the body than the SALT.

French paradox: A term given to the observation that in a certain region of France, where the people should have had a high occurrence of cardiovascular disease due to a high fat diet. However, the disease rate was low due to the preventative action of the chemicals in red wine consumed in the region.

frequency: A term used to describe the position of a peak in SPECTROSCOPY. Frequency is proportional to the ENERGY in ELECTROMAGNETIC RADIATION which is responsible for such peaks. Also, the number of periods occurring in a WAVE in a fixed amount of time.

functional group: A collection of ATOMS bound together in a specific way; also the focal point of most reactions and intermolecular attractions.

GC-MS: Gas chromatograph-mass spectrometer. A two-part instrument; the gas chromatograph performs a separation, and the mass spectrometer can be used for identification and quantification.

genus: A taxonomical group one level above species and one level below family. Plants in the same genus have many similarities including the biochemistry that leads to the production of MOLECULES of medicinal interest.

geometry: A term referring to the shape of a MOLECULE.

glycoprotein: A protein in which some of the side chains have sugars attached.

glycoside: A MOLECULE composed of a sugar connected to a small molecule called the AGLYCONE.

gum: One type of complex polysaccharide; often used as a food additive.

HPLC: High performance (or high pressure) liquid chromatograph. An instrument which performs separations and/or analysis of mixtures using COLUMN CHROMATOGRAPHY.

hydrocarbon: A MOLECULE containing only carbon and hydrogen.

hydrogen bond: An attraction between a hydrogen atom on an ELECTRONEGATIVE ATOM, such as N or O, and another electron-rich ATOM such as N or O. Terribly misnamed, it is not a BOND but rather a fairly strong attraction.

hydrolysis: A reaction in which a MOLECULE is broken down by the addition of water.

hydrophobic: Something which "fears" water, such as a nonpolar MOLECULE.

immune system: A bodily system that protects against invading organisms.

in vitro: "In glass"; refers to a process occurring in a controlled, nonbiological environment, such as in a test tube.

in vivo: "In life"; refers to a process occurring in natural biological systems.

index of hydrogen deficiency (IHD): A measure of how many hydrogen ATOMS are missing from a MOLECULE compared to the corresponding SATURATED HYDROCARBON. One IHD represents two fewer hydrogens than the analogous SATURATED molecule.

inert gas: An ELEMENT in the helium family, found in the eighteenth column of the PERIODIC TABLE; considered very unreactive. Also referred to as the Noble Gases.

inflammation: Redness and swelling due to the reaction of the body to foreign substances or localized damage.

infrared spectroscopy: An instrumental method in which a MOLECULE absorbs infrared radiation. The particular frequencies absorbed can give clues about the FUNCTIONAL GROUPS present in the molecule.

inhibition: A process in which a MOLECULE, such as an ENZYME, is prevented from carrying out its tasks due to interference from an INHIBITOR.

inhibitor: A comparatively small molecule which inhibits the action of an enzyme. An ANTAGONIST could be considered an inhibitor of a RECEPTOR. An inhibitor might also be considered a LIGAND.

initiation: The first step of a radical reaction wherein the radical is first formed.

insufflation: Snorting a drug into the nasal passages.

intercalation: A mode of binding in which a relatively flat molecule binds to DNA by slipping in between two sets of adjacent base pairs. The molecules are held together largely by LONDON FORCES.

ion: A charged ATOM or MOLECULE.

ion channel: A type of TRANSMEMBRANE PROTEIN RECEPTOR that serves to admit IONS in and out of a cell. The ion channel is typically opened or closed by particular LIGANDS and serves to trigger electrical transmission of nerve impulses.

ionic bond: A BOND created when two ATOMS trade ELECTRONS, and then attract each other due to their opposing charges.

IR: Infrared; One type of ELECTROMAGNETIC RADIATION which is used in INFRARED SPECTROSCOPY to determine the types of FUNCTIONAL GROUPS present in a MOLECULE.

ischemia: A period of reduced blood flow to an organ.

isomers: Most fundamentally, MOLECULES which have the same MOLECULAR FORMULA but differ in their structure. These are STRUCTURAL or CONSTITUTIONAL isomers that differ from one another in their CONNECTIVITY.

isoprene rule: A rule used to determine if a MOLECULE is a terpene. States that terpenes are made from branched five-carbon building blocks similar to the molecule isoprene, and that they are usually formed from head-to-tail combinations of these isoprene units.

isotopes: ATOMS of a particular ELEMENT that differ in the number of NEUTRONS in the NUCLEUS.

isozymes: ISOMERS of enzymes that differ slightly in their affinity for the molecules they act upon.

lactone: A cyclic ester group.

LDL: *See* LOW DENSITY LIPOPROTEIN.

Lewis Structure: A symbolic representation of an atom, consisting of the ATOMIC SYMBOL surrounded by the VALENCE ELECTRONS, which are represented by dots.

ligand: A comparatively small MOLECULE that binds to a RECEPTOR or another, larger molecule, and elicits a response. The ligand does not undergo a chemical change. Compare to SUBSTRATE.

linear: A MOLECULAR SHAPE created when a central atom is surrounded by two groups of ELECTRONS, having BOND ANGLES of 180°.

lipid: A class of very nonpolar or hydrophobic MOLECULES.

lipid bilayer: An arrangement of LIPID MOLECULES in which the nonpolar tails point toward each other, and the polar head groups are oriented toward the external water environment. The result is a sandwichlike organization with a nonpolar "filling" and polar "bread."

liquid chromatography: A form of CHROMATOGRAPHY in which the MOBILE PHASE is a liquid.

London forces: Weak attractions between MOLECULES that are most important in nonpolar molecules. London forces are the basis for hydrophobicity, which is a way of saying that nonpolar molecules "fear" water, a polar molecule.

low density lipoprotein (LDL): A particle in the blood that is composed of lipids and a protein called apoB.

macrophage: A circulating immune cell that ingests and destroys foreign bodies which invade the body.

magnetic resonance imaging: A body imaging technique that works on the principles of NMR.

mass spectrometer: An instrument that measures the mass of MOLECULES.

membrane: A LIPID BILAYER that surrounds a cell and provides a barrier between the cell and the outside world.

metabolism: The chemical reactions which serve to break down or create molecules in the body.

microtubules: Tubular structures in cells that are generally only visible during MITOSIS. Composed primarily of two PROTEINS called α- and β-tubulin.

mitochondrion: An structure within a cell (an organelle) responsible for generating ENERGY by breaking down glucose.

mitosis: The process of cell division.

mobile phase: The SOLVENT or gas in a CHROMATOGRAPHY experiment that moves through or over the STATIONARY PHASE and carries dissolved MOLECULES along.

molecular formula: A list of the ELEMENTS and their amounts present in a MOLECULE. Usually listed in the order C, H, and any other atoms alphabetically, in honor of carbon's great importance!

molecular shape: The shape of a MOLECULE; also called the GEOMETRY.

molecule: A combination of two or more ATOMS with a defined CONNECTIVITY.

moment: *See* DIPOLE MOMENT.

MRI: *See* MAGNETIC RESONANCE IMAGING.

MS: *See* MASS SPECTROMETER.

mutation: A change in the base sequence of DNA from normal.

necrosis: Cell death and tissue damage resulting from disease processes or damage; generally mediated by ROS. Compare to APOPTOSIS.

neurotransmission: The release of a chemical into a synapse. The chemical transmission of a nerve impulse between two cells.

neutralize: The process of reacting acidic or basic solutions or MOLECULES so that they become neutral.

neutron: A subatomic particle which has no charge and which is found in the NUCLEUS of an atom.

Newman projection: A view of a MOLECULE looking down or along a BOND.

NMR: Nuclear magnetic resonance. A instrumental method of studying structure based upon the magnetic behavior of the NUCLEUS.

Noble Gas: *See* INERT GAS.

nucleus: The central core of an atom, composed of PROTONS and usually NEUTRONS.

octet rule: A rule that states that ATOMS will try to have eight ELECTRONS in their valence ORBITALS for stability.

ointment: A cream or oily carrier containing medicine.

orbital: A region of space around the NUCLEUS in which an ELECTRON is likely to be found.

outer shell electron: *See* VALENCE ELECTRON.

oxidation: A reaction that adds oxygen ATOMS to a MOLECULE (more strictly, a reaction in which ELECTRONS are lost from a molecule).

oxidative burst: *See* RESPIRATORY BURST.

oxidative stress: The situation in which damage to biomolecules by ROS exceeds the ability of the system to repair itself, resulting in the accumulation of damaged biomolecules.

oxyradical: Another term for REACTIVE OXYGEN SPECIES.

parasympathetic nervous system: The part of the involuntary nervous system that controls digestion, energy storage, bodily rest, and repair. Compare to the SYMPATHETIC NERVOUS SYSTEM.

partial charge: A noninteger charge that results from the uneven sharing of ELECTRONS in a COVALENT BOND, which in turn is due to differences in ELECTRONEGATIVITY between two bonded ATOMS.

peptide: A short chain of about two to fifty or so amino acids. Any longer and the molecule should be called a PROTEIN.

periodic table: A table containing all the elements organized into columns and rows based on their properties and reactions. The basis for the table is the ELECTRON CONFIGURATION.

pH: A measure of the acidity or basicity of a solution. Ultimately related to the number of PROTONS present in a solution.

phagocyte: A circulating immune cell that ingests and dissolves foreign proteins, bacteria, and viruses which invade the body.

phagocytosis: The process by which a cell surrounds and ingests foreign material.

pharmacognosy: The study of all aspects of natural medicinal substances.

pharmacokinetics: The study of how fast a drug is absorbed, distributed, and excreted from the body.

pharmacology: The study of drugs and their effects.

phenyl group: A benzene ring connected to something by a single BOND. Often abbreviated Ph; don't confuse with pH.

photoreactive: A term describing a MOLECULE that can undergo a reaction when it interacts with light (ELECTROMAGNETIC RADIATION).

physiology: The study of the function of organs and whole organisms.

platelet aggregation: Part of the process of blood clotting.

polarity: The property of a MOLECULE arising from the separation of charge within it.

polymer: A long chain of repeating molecular units.

polymerase: An ENZYME that synthesizes a biological POLYMER.

primary metabolism: MOLECULES and processes necessary for life.

primary ROS: The first ROS formed by a biological process, which gives rise to all other ROS.

propagation: The second stage of a radical reaction characterized by a CHAIN REACTION.

protease: An ENZYME that cuts apart proteins.

protein: A long chain of amino acids that folds into a functional unit.

protein backbone: The long chain of ATOMS that forms the structural framework of a PROTEIN.

proton: A positively charged subatomic particle found in the NUCLEUS of an atom. In an acid-base reaction, a proton is the ACID.

qualitative analysis: An analysis of a mixture of MOLECULES designed to identify how many different molecules are in the mixture, and to identify the molecules.

quantitative analysis: An analysis of a mixture of MOLECULES designed to give information about how much of each molecule is present. Generally a QUALITATIVE ANALYSIS must precede a quantitative analysis.

quantum mechanics: A theory involving both physics and chemistry that studies the behavior of ELECTRONS.

R: A symbolic placeholder used in chemical structures to represent a generic portion of a MOLECULE; often denotes a carbon atom attached to other unspecified ATOMS.

racemic mixture: A 50:50 mixture of ENANTIOMERS.

radiation: Light or ELECTROMAGNETIC RADIATION. Also, the emission of rays or particles usually from an atom's NUCLEUS.

radical: A MOLECULE with an unpaired ELECTRON. See also CAGED RADICAL and FREE RADICAL.

rate of reaction: The speed at which a chemical reaction occurs.

reactive oxygen species (ROS): A MOLECULE containing oxygen in a reactive form.

reactivity: The propensity of a MOLECULE to react with another molecule. A highly reactive molecule is not very selective about what it reacts with.

receptor: A structurally complex protein which can bind with a messenger MOLECULE or LIGAND. Upon binding, some sort of action or response occurs.

reductionism: The practice of scientists who try to reduce something to its basic parts so as to gain a better understanding of it and how it works.

reference spectrum: An authentic SPECTRUM of a MOLECULE which can be compared to an unknown spectrum in the hopes of identifying the unknown molecule.

respiratory burst: A sudden increase in the consumption of oxygen by a PHAGOCYTE after it engulfs a foreign cell. The oxygen is converted to ROS.

RNA: Ribonucleic acid; the secondary genetic material responsible for carrying the information in DNA to the cellular machinery which makes proteins.

ROS: *See* REACTIVE OXYGEN SPECIES.

salt: An ionic compound formed when an ACID and a BASE react.

SAR: See STRUCTURE-ACTIVITY RELATIONSHIP.

saturated: A MOLECULE that contains only single BONDS and therefore has as many hydrogen ATOMS as possible.

sawhorse view: A perspective view of a MOLECULE designed to show the particular CONFORMATION.

secondary metabolism: The MOLECULES and processes not required for the short-term functioning of an organism.

selectivity: The propensity of a MOLECULE to react only with other molecules which are either more or less reactive. A highly selective molecule is not very reactive.

semisynthesis: Using a MOLECULE found in nature as a starting point for the synthesis of another molecule, generally of superior medical and toxicological qualities.

separatory funnel: A piece of glassware designed to make liquid-liquid EXTRACTIONS easier by making the interface between the two liquid layers more visible.

side chain: The ATOMS and FUNCTIONAL GROUPS attached to a PROTEIN backbone.

soluble: A term describing a MOLECULE that will dissolve in a given SOLVENT.

solute: A substance that is dissolved in a SOLVENT to form a solution.

solvent: A substance, usually liquid, in which the SOLUTE is dissolved to form a solution.

spectroscopy: The use of light and its interaction with MOLECULES to determine the structure of the molecules or the quantity of the molecules present.

spectrum: Any specific range of ELECTROMAGNETIC RADIATION.

stationary phase: A solid or semisolid material in a CHROMATOGRAPHY experiment which may attract molecules dissoved in the MOBILE PHASE. It is called stationary because it is arranged in the apparatus so that it does not move, while the MOBILE PHASE flows over or through it.

structural isomers: MOLECULES that have the same MOLECULAR FORMULA but different CONNECTIVITIES.

structure-activity relationship (SAR): A relationship between the structure of a MOLECULE and its biological activity. The relationship is generally seen as small changes are made in a structure which in turn vary the biological activity. The use of SAR is one way to improve the usefulness of a drug, by increasing the desired effects and decreasing side effects.

substrate: A comparatively small MOLECULE which binds to an ENZYME and undergoes a chemical reaction. Compare to LIGAND.

sulfhydryl: see THIOL.

supercoiling: The process of coiling the DNA double helix even further to compact long pieces of DNA so that they will fit in the cell.

symmetry: A characteristic of some MOLECULES in which one portion of the structure is identical to another, and the parts are related by rotation around an axis or reflection in a mirror plane.

sympathetic nervous system: The part of the involuntary nervous system that reacts to danger and fear, preparing the body for fight or flight. Compare to the PARASYMPATHETIC NERVOUS SYSTEM.

synapse: The gap between two neurons through which the nerve impulse travels chemically, by NEUROTRANSMISSION.

systematic nomenclature: A highly organized method chemists use to name chemicals.

target: The site of action of a drug on a molecular level.

termination: The final stage of a radical reaction in which the reaction stops due to the annihilation of radicals by their reaction with each other.

tetrahedron: A MOLECULAR SHAPE created when a central atom is surrounded by four groups of ELECTRONS, having BOND ANGLES of 109.5°.

therapeutic margin: The difference between the toxic and the therapeutic dose of a chemical substance.

thioglycoside: A GLYCOSIDE in which the sugar portion and the AGLYCONE are connected by a sulfur atom.

thiol: A functional group containing the ATOMS –SH; similar to an alcohol.

tincture: A plant EXTRACT prepared in alcohol.

TLC: Thin layer CHROMATOGRAPHY.

topoisomerase: A class of ENZYMES which affect the degree of SUPERCOILING of DNA by either winding or unwinding the supercoils.

toxic oxygen free radical: See REACTIVE OXYGEN SPECIES.

toxicology: The study of toxic substances and their effects.

trade name: A common name for a drug, typically trademarked.

trans: A term referring to the arrangement of groups on a double BOND in which the major or largest groups on each end of the double BOND are on opposite sides. Compare to *CIS*.

transmembrane protein: A PROTEIN molecule embedded in a MEMBRANE and which spans the entire membrane.

trigonal planar: A MOLECULAR SHAPE in which a central atom is surrounded by three groups of ELECTRONS, having BOND ANGLES of 120°.

unsaturated: A MOLECULE that contains double and/or triple BONDS, and therefore does not have as many hydrogen ATOMS as its SATURATED relative.

valence electron: An ELECTRON in one of the outer or bonding ORBITALS of an atom.

vector: An arrow carrying information about both direction and magnitude of a quantity.

vesicle: A small "container" within a cell which is used to store molecules of particular types.

visualization method: One of a variety of techniques, such as the use of ultraviolet light, to see compounds otherwise invisible to the human eye.

VSEPR theory: Valence shell electron pair repulsion theory, which states that the MOLECULAR SHAPE can be predicted based upon the repulsion of groups of ELECTRONS around a central atom.

wave: A disturbance or vibration moving through a medium, such as air or water, or an analogous variation in a magnetic or electric field.

wavelength: The distance between two consecutive troughs or crests of a WAVE.

wavenumber: A unit of measure used in IR SPECTROSCOPY, written cm^{-1}.

xenobiotic: A molecule not normally found in the body. Compare to ENDOGENOUS.

zoopharmacognosy: The study of how animals use medicinally active plants.

Bibliography

Agosta, William C. (1997). Medicines and drugs from plants. *Journal of Chemical Education* 74: 857-860.

Ahlemeyer, Barbara and Josef Krieglstein (1998). Neuroprotective effects of *Ginkgo biloba* extract. In Larry D. Lawson and Rudolf Bauer (eds.), *Phytomedicines of Europe: Chemistry and biological activity* (pp. 210-220). Washington, DC: American Chemical Society.

Airaksinen, Mauno M., Heikki Svensk, Jouko Tuomisto, and Hannu Komulainen (1980). Tetrahydro-β-carbolines and corresponding tryptamines: In vitro inhibition of serotonin and dopamine uptake by human blood platelets. *Acta Pharmacologica et Toxicologica* 46: 308-313.

Ames, Bruce N., Mark K. Shigenaga, and Tory M. Hagen (1993). Oxidants, antioxidants, and the degenerative diseases of aging. *Proceedings of the National Academy of Science USA* 90: 7915-7922.

Ashok, Badithe T. and Rashid Ali (1999). The aging paradox: Free radical theory of aging. *Experimental Gerontology* 34: 293-303.

Atta-Ur-Rahman, Azra Pervin, and M. Iqbal Choudhary (1991). Sophazrine—A novel quinolizidine alkaloid from *Sophora griffithii. Journal of Natural Products* 54: 929-935.

Bailly, Christian (2000). Topoisomerase I poisons and suppressors as anticancer drugs. *Current Medicinal Chemistry* 7: 39-58.

Barbieri, Luigi, Maria Giulia Battelli, and Fiorenzo Stirpe (1993). Ribosome-inactivating proteins from plants. *Biochimica et Biophysica Acta* 1154: 237-282.

Bisset, Norma G. (1995). Arrow poisons and their role in the development of medicinal agents. In Richard Evans Schultes and Siri Von Reis (eds.), *Ethnobotany: Evolution of a discipline* (pp. 289-302). Portland, OR: Dioscorides Press.

Block, Gladys, Blossom Patterson, and Amy Subar (1992). Fruit, vegetables, and cancer prevention: A review of the epidemiological evidence. *Nutrition and Cancer* 18: 1-29.

Blumenthal, Mark (2003). *The ABC clinical guide to herbs.* New York: American Botanical Council.

Blumenthal, Mark, Alicia Goldberg, and Josef Brinkmann (2000). *Herbal medicine: Expanded Commission E monographs.* Newton, MA: Integrative Medicine Communications.

Bonson, Katherine R., Joshua W. Buckholtz, and Dennis L. Murphy (1996). Chronic administration of serotonergic antidepressants attenuates the subjective effects of LSD in humans. *Neuropsychopharmacology* 16: 425-436.

Bonson, Katherine R. and Dennis L. Murphy (1996). Alterations in response to LSD in humans associated with chronic administration of tricyclic antidepressants, monoamine oxidase inhibitors or lithium. *Behavioural Brain Research* 73: 229-233.

Botta, Bruno, Giuliano Delle Monache, Domenico Misiti, Alberto Vitali, and Giovanni Zappia (2001). Aryltetralin lignans: Chemistry, pharmacology and biotransformations. *Current Medicinal Chemistry* 8: 1363-1381.

Braquet, P. and J.J. Godfroid (1987). Conformational properties of the PAF-acether receptor on platelets based on structure-activity studies. In Fred Snyder (ed.), *Platelet-activating factor and related lipid mediators* (pp. 191-235). New York: Plenum Press.

Braquet, P., L. Touqui, T.Y. Shen, and B.B. Vargaftig (1987). Perspectives in platelet-activating factor research. *Pharmacological Reviews* 39: 97-145.

Braquet, Pierre (1986). Proofs of involvement of PAF-acether in various immune disorders using BN 52021 (Ginkgolide B): A powerful PAF-acether antagonist isolated from *Ginkgo biloba* L. In U. Zor, Z. Naor, and F. Kohen (eds.), *Advances in prostaglandin, thromboxane, and leukotriene research,* Volume 16 (pp. 179-198). New York: Raven Press.

Bruneton, Jean (1995). *Pharmacognosy, phytochemistry, medicinal plants.* Paris, France: Lavoisier Publishing.

Burcham, Philip C. (1999). Internal hazards: Baseline DNA damage by endogenous products of normal metabolism. *Mutation Research* 443: 11-36.

Burris, Kevin D., Marsha B. Reeding, and Elaine Sanders-Bush (1991). (+)Lysergic acid diethylamide, but not its nonhallucinogenic congeners, is a potent serotonin $5HT_{1C}$ receptor agonist. *The Journal of Pharmacology and Experimental Therapeutics* 258: 891-896.

Callaway, James C., Mauno M. Airaksinen, Dennis J. McKenna, Glacus S. Brito, and Charles S. Grob (1994). Platelet serotonin uptake sites increased in drinkers of ayahuasca. *Psychopharmacology* 116: 385-387.

Callaway, J.C. and D.J. McKenna (1998). Neurochemistry of psychedelic drugs. In Steven B. Karch (ed.), *Drug abuse handbook* (pp. 485-498). Boca Raton, FL: CRC Press.

Callaway, J.C., D.J. McKenna, C.S. Grob, G.S. Brito, L.P. Raymon, R.E. Poland, E.N. Andrade, E.O. Andrade, and D.C. Mash (1999). Pharmacokinetics of *Hoasca* alkaloids in healthy humans. *Journal of Ethnopharmacology* 65: 243-256.

Carr, Anitra C., Mark R. McCall, and Balz Frei (2000). Oxidation of LDL by myeloperoxidase and reactive nitrogen species: Reaction pathways and antioxidant protection. *Arteriosclerosis, Thrombosis, and Vascular Biology* 10: 1716-1723.

Chang, Tsu-Chung, Wei-Yuan Chou, and Gu-Gang Chang (2000). Protein oxidation and turnover. *Journal of Biomedical Science* 7: 357-363.

Charlton, James L. (1998). Antiviral activity of lignans. *Journal of Natural Products* 61: 1447-1451.

Chavez, Mary L. and Pedro I. Chavez (1998). Ginkgo (part 1): History, use and pharmacologic properties. *Hospital Pharmacy* 33: 658-672.

Chen, Juan Juan and Byung Pal Yu (1994). Alterations in mitochondrial membrane fluidity by lipid peroxidation products. *Free Radical Biology & Medicine* 17: 411-418.

Chisolm III, Guy M., Stanley L. Hazen, Paul L. Fox, and Martha K. Cathcart (1999). The oxidation of lipoproteins by monocytes-macrophages. *The Journal of Biological Chemistry* 274: 25959-25962.

Choe, Myeon, Christ Jackson, and Byung Pal Yu (1995). Lipid peroxidation contributes to age-related membrane rigidity. *Free Radical Biology & Medicine* 18: 977-984.

Cichewicz, Robert H. and Patrick A. Thorpe (1996). The antimicrobial properties of chile peppers (*Capsicum* species) and their uses in Mayan medicine. *Journal of Ethnopharmacology* 52: 61-70.

Curzio, Marina (1988). Interaction between neutrophils and 4-hydroxyalkenals and consequences on neutrophil motility. *Free Radical Research Communications* 5: 55-66.

Damayanthi, Yalamati and J. William Lown (1998). Podophyllotoxins: Current status and recent developments. *Current Medicinal Chemistry* 5: 205-252.

Dassonneville, Laurent, Amelie Lansiaux, Aurelie Wattelet, Nicole Wattez, Christine Mahieu, Sabine Van Miert, Luc Pieters, and Christian Bailly (2000). Cytotoxicity and cell cycle effects of the plant alkaloids cryptolepine and neocryptolepine: Relation to drug induced apoptosis. *European Journal of Pharmacology* 409: 9-18.

Davies, Michael J., Shanlin Fu, Hongjie Wang, and Roger T. Dean (1999). Stable markers of oxidant damage to proteins and their application in the study of human disease. *Free Radical Biology & Medicine* 27: 1151-1163.

Deliganis, Anna V., Pamela A. Pierce, and Stephen J. Peroutka (1991). Differential interactions of dimethyltryptamine (DMT) with 5-HT_{1A} and 5-HT_2 receptors. *Biochemical Pharmacology* 41: 1739-1744.

Deng, Jing-Zhen, Shelley R. Starck, and Sidney M. Hecht (1999). DNA polymerase β inhibitors from *Baeckea gunniana*. *Journal of Natural Products* 62: 1624-1626.

Deng, Jing-Zhen, Shelley R. Starck, and Sidney M. Hecht (2000). Pentacyclic triterpenoids from *Freziera* sp. that inhibit DNA polymerase β. *Bioorganic & Medicinal Chemistry* 8: 247-250.

Desai, Arshad and Timothy J. Mitchison (1997). Microtubule polymerization dynamics. *Annual Review of Cell and Developmental Biology* 13: 83-117.

Dobretsov, G.E., T.A. Borschevskaya, V.A. Petrov, and Y.A. Vladimirov (1977). The increase of phospholipid bilayer rigidity after lipid peroxidation. *FEBS Letters* 84: 125-128.

Dostal, Jiri (2000). Two faces of alkaloids. *Journal of Chemical Education* 77: 993-998.

Downing, Kenneth H. (2000). Structural basis for the interaction of tubulin with proteins and drugs that affect microtubule dynamics. *Annual Review of Cell and Developmental Biology* 16: 89-111.

Dukan, S., A. Farewell, M. Ballesteros, F. Taddei, M. Radman, and T. Nystrom (2000). Protein oxidation in response to increased transcriptional or translational errors. *Proceedings of the National Academy of Science USA* 97: 5746-5749.

Dumontet, Charles (2000). Mechanisms of action and resistance to tubulin-binding agents. *Expert Opinion Investigational Drugs* 9: 779-788.

Eze, M.O. (1992). Membrane fluidity, reactive oxygen species, and cell-mediated immunity: Implications in nutrition and disease. *Medical Hypotheses* 37: 220-224.

Fiorella, D., R.A. Rabin, and J.C. Winter (1995a). The role of the 5-HT_{2A} and 5-HT_{2C} receptors in the stimulus effects of hallucinogenic drugs I: Antagonist correlation analysis. *Psychopharmacology* 121: 347-356.

Fiorella, D., R.A. Rabin, and J.C. Winter (1995b). Role of 5-HT_{2A} and 5-HT_{2C} receptors in the stimulus effects of hallucinogenic drugs II: Reassessment of LSD false positives. *Psychopharmacology* 121: 357-363.

Frankel, E.N., J. Kanner, J.B. German, E. Parks, and J.E. Kinsella (1993). Inhibition of oxidation of human low-density lipoprotein by phenolic substances in red wine. *The Lancet* 341: 454-457.

Frankel, Edwin N., Andrew L. Waterhouse, and Pierre L. Teissedre (1995). Principal phenolic phytochemicals in selected California wines and their antioxidant activity inhibiting oxidation of human low-density lipoproteins. *Journal of Agricultural and Food Chemistry* 43: 890-894.

Fulda, Simone, Carsten Scaffidi, Santos A. Susin, Peter H. Krammer, Guido Kroemer, Marcus E. Peter, and Klaus-Michael Debatin (1998). Activation of mitochondria and release of mitochondrial apoptogenic factors by betulinic acid. *The Journal of Biological Chemistry* 273: 33942-33948.

Gamet-Payrastre, Laurence, Pengfei Li, Solange Lumeau, Georges Cassar, Marie-Ange Dupont, Sylvie Chevolleau, Nicole Gasc, Jacques Tulliez, and Francois Terce (2000). Sulforaphane, a naturally occurring isothiocyanate, induces cell cycle arrest and apoptosis in HT29 human colon cancer cells. *Cancer Research* 60: 1426-1433.

Garcia-Carbonero, Rocio and Jeffrey G. Supko (2002). Current perspectives on the clinical experience, pharmacology, and continued development of the camptothecins. *Clinical Cancer Research* 8: 641-661.

Glennon, Richard A., Mikhail Bondarev, and Bryan Roth (1999). 5-HT_6 serotonin receptor binding of indolealkylamines: A preliminary structure-affinity investigation. *Medicinal Chemistry Research* 9: 108-117.

Glennon, Richard A., Malgorzata Dukat, Mohamed El-Bermawy, Ho Law, Joseph De Los Angeles, Milt Teitler, Allison King, and Katherine Herrick-Davis (1994).

Influence of amine substituents on 5-HT$_{2A}$ versus 5-HT$_{2C}$ binding of phenyl-alkyl- and indolylalkylamines. *Journal of Medicinal Chemistry* 37: 1929-1935.

Glennon, Richard A., Malgorzata Dukat, Brian Grella, Seoung-Soo Hong, Luca Costantino, Milt Teitler, Carol Smith, Chris Egan, Katherine Davis, and Mariena V. Mattson (2000). Binding of β-carbolines and related agents at serotonin (5-HT$_2$ and 5-HT$_{1A}$), dopamine (D$_2$) and benzodiazepine receptors. *Drug and Alcohol Dependence* 60: 121-132.

Glennon, Richard A., Mase Lee, Jagadeesh B. Rangisetty, Malgorzata Dukat, Bryan L. Roth, Jason E. Savage, Ace McBride, Laura Rauser, Sandy Hufeisen, and David K.H. Lee (2000). 2-Substituted tryptamines: Agents with selectivity for 5-HT$_6$ serotonin receptors. *Journal of Medicinal Chemistry* 43: 1011-1018.

Glennon, Richard A., Milt Titeler, and J.D. McKenney (1984). Evidence for 5-HT$_2$ involvement in the mechanism of action of hallucinogenic agents. *Life Sciences* 35: 2505-2511.

Gordaliza, M., M.A. Castro, J.M. Miguel del Corral, and A. San Feliciano (2000). Antitumor properties of podophyllotoxin and related compounds. *Current Pharmaceutical Design* 6: 1811-1839.

Greenwood, David (1992). The quinine connection. *Journal of Antimicrobial Chemotherapy* 30: 417-427.

Grella, Brian, Malgorzata Dukat, Richard Young, Milt Teitler, Katherine Herrick-Davis, Colleen B. Gauthier, and Richard A. Glennon (1998). Investigation of hallucinogenic and related β-carbolines. *Drug and Alcohol Dependence* 50: 99-107.

Haslam, Edwin (1995). Natural polyphenols (vegetable tannins) as drugs: Possible modes of action. *Journal of Natural Products* 59: 205-215.

Hatefi, Youssef and Dianna L. Stiggall (1976). Succinate dehydrogenases. In Paul D. Boyer (ed.), *The enzymes,* Volume XIII: *Oxidation-reduction Part C dehydrogenases (II) oxidases (II) hydrogen peroxide cleavage,* Third edition (pp. 222-257). New York: Academic Press.

Hecht, Stephen S. (1999). Chemoprevention of cancer by isothiocyanates, modifiers of carcinogen metabolism. *Journal of Nutrition* 1: 768S-774S.

Helsley, Scott, David Fiorella, Richard A. Rabin, and J.C. Winter (1998). A comparison of N,N-dimethyltryptamine, harmaline, and selected congeners in rats trained with LSD as a discriminative stimulus. *Progress in Neuro-Psychopharmacology & Biological Psychiatry* 22: 649-663.

Hertog, Michael G.L., Edith J.M. Feskens, Peter C.H. Hollman, Martijn B. Katan, and Dean Kromhout (1993). Dietary antioxidant flavonoids and risk of coronary heart disease: The Zutphen Elderly Study. *The Lancet* 342: 1007-1011.

Hertzberg, Robert P., Mary Jo Caranfa, and Sidney M. Hecht (1989). On the mechanism of topoisomerase I inhibition by camptothecin: Evidence for binding to an enzyme-DNA complex. *Biochemistry* 28: 4629-4638.

Hesse, Manfred (2002). *Alkaloids: Nature's curse or blessing?* Weinheim, Germany: Wiley-VCH.

Hong, S., M. Dukat, M. Teitler, C. Egan, A. Dupre, K. Herrick-Davis, and R.A. Glennon (1999). 5,8-Dimethoxyharmalan: Actions at 5-HT$_{2A}$ serotonin receptors. *Medicinal Chemistry Research* 9: 374-388.

Houghton, Peter J. (2001). Old yet new—Pharmaceuticals from plants. *Journal of Chemical Education* 78: 175-184.

Hoyer, D. and G. Martin (1997). 5-HT Receptor classification and nomenclature: Towards a harmonization with the human genome. *Neuropharmacology* 36: 419-428.

Ismaiel, Abd M., Kim Arruda, Milt Teitler, and Richard A. Glennon (1995). Ketanserin analogues: The effect of structural modification on 5-HT$_2$ serotonin receptor binding. *Journal of Medicinal Chemistry* 38: 1196-1202.

Iverson, Tina M., Cesar Luna-Chavez, Gary Cecchini, and Douglas C. Rees (1999). Structure of the *Escherichia coli* fumarate reductase respiratory complex. *Science* 284: 1961-1966.

Jacobs, Barry L. (1987). How hallucinogenic drugs work. *American Scientist* 75: 386-392.

Kehrer, Diederik F.S., Otto Soepenberg, Walter J. Loos, Jaap Verweij, and Alex Sparreboom (2001). Modulation of camptothecin analogs in the treatment of cancer: A review. *Anti-Cancer Drugs* 12: 89-105.

Kehrer, James P. (1993). Free radicals as mediators of tissue injury and disease. *Critical Reviews in Toxicology* 23: 21-48.

Knight, Joseph A. (2000). Free radicals, antioxidants, and the immune system. *Annals of Clinical & Laboratory Science* 30: 145-158.

Koltai, Matyas, David Hosford, Philippe Guinot, Andre Esanu, and Pierre Braquet (1991a). PAF: A review of its effects, antagonists and possible future clinical implications (part I). *Drugs* 42: 9-29.

Koltai, Matyas, David Hosford, Philippe Guinot, Andre Esanu, and Pierre Braquet (1991b). PAF: A review of its effects, antagonists and possible future clinical implications (part II). *Drugs* 42: 174-204.

Kostansek, Edward C., William N. Lipscomb, R. Rogers Yocum, and William E. Thiessen (1978). Conformation of the mushroom toxin β-amanitin in the crystalline state. *Biochemistry* 17: 3790-3795.

Kristiansen, Kurt and Svein G. Dahl (1996). Molecular modeling of serotonin, ketanserin, ritanserin and their 5-HT$_{2C}$ receptor interactions. *European Journal of Pharmacology* 306: 195-210.

Lanni, Jennifer S., Scott W. Lowe, Edward J. Licitra, Jun O. Liu, and Tyler Jacks (1997). P53-independent apoptosis induced by paclitaxel through an indirect mechanism. *Proceedings of the National Academy of Science USA* 94: 9679-9683.

Leathwood, Peter D., Francoise Chauffard, Eva Heck, and Raphael Munoz-Box (1982). Aqueous extract of valerian root (*Valeriana officinalis* L.) improves sleep quality in man. *Pharmacology Biochemistry & Behavior* 17: 65-71.

Lesuisse, D., J. Berjonneau, C. Ciot, P. Devaux, B. Doucet, J.F. Gourvest, B. Khemis, C. Lang, R. Legrand, M. Lowinski, et al. (1996). Determination of oenothein B as the active 5-α-reductase-inhibiting principle of the folk medicine *Epilobium parviflorum. Journal of Natural Products* 59: 490-492.

Li, Tsai-Kun, Eleanor Bathory, Edmond J. LaVoie, A.R. Srinivasan, Wilma K. Olson, Ronald R. Sauers, Leroy F. Liu, and Daniel S. Pilch (2000). Human topoisomerase I poisoning by protoberberines: Potential roles for both drug-DNA and drug-enzyme interactions. *Biochemistry* 39: 7107-7116.

Li, Tsai-Kun and Leroy F. Liu (2001). Tumor cell death induced by topoisomerase-targeting drugs. *Annual Review of Pharmacology and Toxicology* 41: 53-77.

Loft, S. and H.E. Poulson (1996). Cancer risk and oxidative DNA damage in man. *Journal of Molecular Medicine* 74: 297-312.

Lord, J. Michael, Lynne M. Roberts, and Jon D. Robertus (1994). Ricin: Structure, mode of action, and some current applications. *The FASEB Journal* 8: 201-208.

Malkas, Linda H. (1998). DNA replication machinery of the mammalian cell. *Journal of Cellular Biochemistry Supplements* 30/31: 18-29.

Marnett, Lawrence J., Scott W. Rowlinson, Douglas C. Goodwin, Amit S. Kalgutkar, and Cheryl A. Lanzo (1999). Arachidonic acid oxygenation by COX-1 and COX-2. *The Journal of Biological Chemistry* 274: 22903-22906.

McKenna, Dennis J., G.H.N. Towers, and F.S. Abbott (1984a). Monoamine oxidase inhibitors in South American hallucinogenic plants: Tryptamine and β-carboline constituents of ayahuasca. *Journal of Ethnopharmacology* 10: 195-223.

McKenna, Dennis J., G.H.N. Towers, and F.S. Abbott (1984b). Monoamine oxidase inhibitors in South American hallucinogenic plants part 2: Constituents of orally-active myristicaceous hallucinogens. *Journal of Ethnopharmacology* 12: 179-211.

Meert, T.F., P. de Haes, and P.A.J. Johnson (1989). Risperidone (R 64 766), a potent and complete LSD antagonist in drug discrimination by rats. *Psychopharmacology* 97: 206-212.

Metzner, Ralph (1999). *Ayahuasca: Human consciousness and the spirits of nature.* New York: Thunder's Mouth Press.

Michaels, Mark Leo, Christina Cruz, Arthur P. Grollman, and Jeffrey H. Miller (1992). Evidence that MutY and MutM combine to prevent mutations by an oxidatively damaged form of guanine in DNA. *Proceedings of the National Academy of Science USA* 89: 7022-7025.

Mizushina, Yoshiyuki, Akira Iida, Keisuke Ohta, Fuymio Sugawara, and Kengo Sakaguchi (2000). Novel triterpenoids inhibit both DNA polymerase and DNA topoisomerase. *Biochemistry Journal* 350: 757-763.

Monte, Aaron P., Danuta Marona-Lewicka, Nicholas V. Cozzi, David L. Nelson, and David E. Nichols (1995). Conformationally restricted tetrahydro-1-benzoxepin analogs of hallucinogenic phenethylamines. *Medicinal Chemistry Research* 5: 651-663.

Nencini, Paolo (2002). The shaman and the rave party: Social pharmacology of ecstasy. *Substance Use & Misuse* 37: 923-939.

Newberg, Andrew, Abass Alavi, Michael Baime, Michael Pourdehnad, Jill Santanna, and Eugene d'Aquili (2001). The measurement of regional cerebral blood flow during the complex cognitive task of meditation: A preliminary SPECT study. *Psychiatry Research: Neuroimaging Section* 106: 113-133.

Newberg, Andrew and Eugene G. d'Aquili (2000). The neuropsychology of religious and spiritual experience. *Journal of Consciousness Studies* 7: 251-266.

Nogales, Eva, Michael Whittaker, Ronald A. Milligan, and Kenneth H. Downing (1999). High-resolution model of the microtubule. *Cell* 96: 79-88.

Nogales, Eva, Sharon Grayer Wolf, Israr A. Khan, Richard F. Luduena, and Kenneth H. Downing (1995). Structure of tubulin at 6.5A and location of the taxol-binding site. *Nature* 375: 424-427.

Perrine, Daniel M. (1996). *The chemistry of mind-altering drugs: History, pharmacology, and cultural context.* Washington, DC: American Chemical Society.

Pierce, Pamela A. and Stephen J. Peroutka (1989). Hallucinogenic drug interactions with neurotransmitter receptor binding sites in human cortex. *Psychopharmacology* 97: 118-122.

Pietta, Pier-Giorgio (2000). Flavonoids as antioxidants. *Journal of Natural Products* 63: 1035-1042.

Pisha, Emily, Heebyung Chai, Ik-Soo Lee, Tangai E. Chagwedera, Norman R. Farnsworth, Geoffrey A. Cordell, Christopher W.W. Beecher, Harry H.S. Fong, A. Douglas Kinghorn, Daniel M. Brown, et al. (1995). Discovery of betulinic acid as a selective inhibitor of human melanoma that functions by induction of apoptosis. *Nature Medicine* 1: 1046-1051.

Podrez, Eugene A., Husam M. Abu-Soud, and Stanley L. Hazen (2000). Myeloperoxidase-generated oxidants and atherosclerosis. *Free Radical Biology & Medicine* 28: 1717-1725.

Pollmeni, J. and J.P. Reiss (2002). How shamanism and group selection may reveal the origins of schizophrenia. *Medical Hypotheses* 58: 244-248.

Pourquier, Philippe, Li-Ming Ueng, Jolanta Fertala, David Wang, Hyun-Ju Park, John M. Essigmann, Mary-Ann Bjornsti, and Yves Pommier (1999). Induction of reversible complexes between eukaryotic DNA topoisomerase I and DNA-containing oxidative base damage. *The Journal of Biological Chemistry* 274: 8516-8523.

Prescott, Stephen M., Guy A. Zimmerman, Diana M. Stafforini, and Thomas M. McIntyre (2000). Platelet-activating factor and related lipid mediators. *Annual Review of Biochemistry* 69: 419-445.

Redinbo, Matthew R., Lance Stewart, Peter Kuhn, James J. Champous, and Wim G.J. Hol (1998). Crystal structures of human topoisomerase I in covalent and noncovalent complexes with DNA. *Science* 279: 1504-1513.

Rivier, Laurent and Jan-Erik Lindgren (1972). "Ayahuasca," the South American hallucinogenic drink: An ethnobotanical and chemical investigation. *Economic Botany* 26: 101-129.

Robbers, James E. and Varro E. Tyler (1999). *Tyler's herbs of choice: The therapeutic use of phytomedicinals.* Binghamton, NY: The Haworth Herbal Press.

Sadzot, Bernard, Jay M. Baraban, Richard A. Glennon, Robert A. Lyon, Sigrun Leonhardt, Chung-Ren Jan, and Milt Teitler (1989). Hallucinogenic drug interactions at human brain 5-HT$_2$ receptors: Implications for treating LSD-induced hallucinogenesis. *Psychopharmacology* 98: 495-499.

Samuelsen, Anne Berit (2000). The traditional uses, chemical constituents and biological activities of *Plantago major* L.: A review. *Journal of Ethnopharmacology* 71: 1-21.

Samuelsen, Anne Berit, Berit Smestad Paulsen, Jens Kristian Wold, Hanako Otsuka, Haruki Yamada, and Terje Espevik (1995). Isolation and partial characterization of biologically active polysaccharides from *Plantago major* L. *Phytotherapy Research* 9: 211-218.

Sandvig, Kirsten and Bo Van Deurs (1996). Endocytosis, intracellular transport, and cytotoxic action of shiga toxin and ricin. *Physiological Reviews* 76: 949-966.

Sastre, Juan, Federico V. Pallardo, Jose Garcia de la Asuncion, and Jose Vina (2000). Mitochondria, oxidative stress and aging. *Free Radical Research* 32: 189-198.

Sastre, Juan, Federico V. Pallardo, and Jose Vina (2000). Mitochondrial oxidative stress plays a key role in aging and apoptosis. *IUBMB Life* 49: 427-435.

Schmeller, T., B. Latz-Bruning, and M. Wink (1997). Biochemical activities of berberine, palmatine and sanguinarine mediating chemical defence against microorganisms and herbivores. *Phytochemistry* 44: 257-266.

Schultes, Richard Evans and Robert F. Raffauf (1992). *Vine of the soul: Medicine men, their plants and rituals in the Columbian Amazonia.* Santa Fe, NM: Synergetic Press.

Schulz, Volker, Rudolf Hansel, and Varro E. Tyler (2001). Restlessness and sleep disturbances. In Volker Schulz, Rudolf Hansel, and Varro E. Tyler (eds.), *Rational phytotherapy,* Third edition (pp. 73-88). Berlin: Springer.

Sevanian, Alex and Fulvio Ursini (2000). Lipid peroxidation in membranes and low-density lipoproteins: Similarities and differences. *Free Radical Biology & Medicine* 29: 306-311.

Silverman, Julian (1967). Shamans and acute schizophrenia. *American Anthropologist* 69: 21-31.

Smith, Paul F., Karyn Maclennan, and Cynthia L. Darlington (1996). The neuroproperties of the *Ginkgo biloba* leaf: A review of the possible relationship to platelet-activating factor (PAF). *Journal of Ethnopharmacology* 50: 131-139.

Smith, Randy L., Herve Canton, Robert J. Barrett, and Elaine Sanders-Bush (1998). Agonist properties of N,N-dimethyltryptamine at serotonin 5-HT$_{2A}$ and 5-HT$_{2C}$ receptors. *Pharmacology Biochemistry and Behavior* 61: 323-330.

Sorger, Peter K., Max Dobles, Regis Tournebize, and Anthony A. Hyman (1997). Coupling cell division and cell death to microtubule dynamics. *Current Opinion in Cell Biology* 9: 807-814.

Stadtman, Earl R. (1992). Protein oxidation and aging. *Science* 257: 1220-1224.

Strassman, Rick J. and Clifford R. Qualls (1994). Dose-response study of N,N-dimethyltryptamine in humans: I. Neuroendocrine, autonomic, and cardiovascular effects. *Archives of General Psychiatry* 51: 85-97.

Strassman, Rick J., Clifford Qualls, and Laura M. Berg (1996). Differential tolerance to biological and subjective effects of four closely spaced doses of N,N-dimethyltryptamine in humans. *Biological Psychiatry* 39: 784-795.

Strassman, Rick J., Clifford R. Qualls, Eberhard H. Uhlenhuth, and Robert Kellner (1994). Dose-response study of N,N-dimethyltryptamine in humans: II. Subjective effects and preliminary results of a new rating scale. *Archives of General Psychiatry* 51: 98-108.

Teitler, Milt, Cynthia Scheick, Paul Howard, Joseph E. Sullivan III, Tatsunori Iwamura, and Richard A. Glennon (1997). 5-HT$_{5A}$ serotonin receptor binding: A preliminary structure-affinity investigation. *Medicinal Chemistry Research* 7: 207-218.

Terao, Junji (1991). Reactions of lipid hydroperoxides. In Carmen Vigo-Pelfrey (ed.), *Membrane lipid oxidation* (pp. 219-268). Boca Raton, FL: CRC Press.

Van Beek, T.A., E. Bombardelli, P. Morazzoni, and F. Peterlongo (1998). *Ginkgo biloba* L. *Fitoterapia* 69: 195-244.

Vaya, Jacob, Saeed Mahmood, Amiram Goldblum, Michael Aviram, Nina Volkova, Amin Shaalan, Ramadan Musa, and Snait Tamir (2003). Inhibition of LDL oxidation by flavonoids in relation to their structure and calculated enthalpy. *Phytochemistry* 62: 89-99.

Vinson, Joe A., John Proch, and Ligia Zubik (1999). Phenol antioxidant quantity and quality in foods: Cocoa, dark chocolate, and milk chocolate. *Journal of Agricultural and Food Chemistry* 47: 4821-4824.

Vlietinck, A.J., T. De Bruyne, and D.A. Vanden Berghe (1997). Plant substances as antiviral agents. *Current Organic Chemistry* 1: 307-344.

Wall, Monroe E. and Mansukh C. Wani (1996). Camptothecin and taxol: From discovery to clinic. *Journal of Ethnopharmacology* 51: 239-254.

Wall, Monroe E., M.C. Wani, C.E. Cook, and Keith H. Palmer (1966). Plant antitumor agents: I. The isolation and structure of camptothecin, a novel alkaloidal leukemia and tumor inhibitor from *Camptotheca acuminata*. *Journal of the American Chemical Society* 88: 3888-3890.

Wang, James C. (1996). DNA topoisomerases. *Annual Review of Biochemistry* 65: 635-692.

Watanabe, Coran M.H., Siegfried Wolffram, Peter Ader, Gerald Rimbach, Lester Packer, John J. Maguire, Peter G. Schultz, and Kishorchandra Gohil (2001). The in vivo neuromodulatory effects of the herbal medicine *Ginkgo biloba*. *Proceedings of the National Academy of Science USA* 98: 6577-6580.

Weil, Andrew T. and Wade Davis (1994). *Bufo alvarius:* A potent hallucinogen of animal origin. *Journal of Ethnopharmacology* 41: 1-8.

Wienties, Frans B. and Anthony W. Segal (1995). NADPH oxidase and the respiratory burst. *Cell Biology* 6: 357-365.

Wink, Michael (1998). Modes of action of alkaloids. In M.F. Roberts and Michael Wink (eds.), *Alkaloids: Biochemistry, ecology, and medicinal applications* (pp. 301-326). New York: Plenum Press.

Winter, J.C., R.A. Filipink, D. Timineri, S.E. Helsley, and R.A. Rabin (2000). The paradox of 5-methoxy-N,N-dimethyltryptamine: An indoleamine hallucinogen that induces stimulus control via 5-HT$_{1A}$ receptors. *Pharmacology Biochemistry and Behavior* 65: 75-82.

Wright, Peggy Ann (1989). The nature of the shamanic state of consciousness: A review. *Journal of Psychoactive Drugs* 21: 25-33.

Wu, Jiaxi, Ming-Biao Yin, Gunnar Hapke, Karoly Toth, and Youcef M. Rustum (2002). Induction of biphasic DNA double strand breaks and activation of multiple repair protein complexes by DNA topoisomerase I drug 7-ethyl-10-hydroxy-camptothecin. *Molecular Pharmacology* 61: 742-748.

Xie, Hong-Guang, Richard B. Kim, Alastair J.J. Wood, and C. Michael Stein (2001). Molecular basis of ethnic differences in drug disposition and response. *Annual Review Pharmacology and Toxicology* 41: 815-850.

Yang, Li-Xi, Xiandao Pan, and Hui-Juan Wang (2002). Novel camptothecin derivatives. Part 1: Oxyalkanoic acid esters of camptothecin and their in vitro and in vivo antitumor activity. *Bioorganic & Medicinal Chemistry Letters* 12: 1241-1244.

Zimmerman, Guy A., Thomas M. McIntyre, Meena Mehra, and Stephen M. Prescott (1990). Endothelial cell-associated platelet-activating factor: A novel mechanism for signaling intercellular adhesion. *The Journal of Cell Biology* 110: 529-540.

Zollner, Helmward, Rudolf Jorg Schaur, and Hermann Esterbauer (1991). Biological activities of 4-hydroxyalkenals. In Helmut Sies (ed.), *Oxidative stress: Oxidants and antioxidants* (pp. 337-369). San Diego: Academic Press.

Index